Saw palmetto

THE HERB FOR PROSTATE HEALTH

Christopher Hobbs, L.AC. *and*
Stephen Brown, N.D.

In this book, the author is not prescribing herbs or other substances for any medical condition, but rather describing their historical and current use. The material in this book is not a substitute for individual advice from your health-care practitioner. The author and editors of this book emphasize that a total program for health, which can often effectively include an herbal regimen, is the only lasting and sure way to assist the body in its healing processes.

Saw Palmetto: The Herb for Prostate Health
Christopher Hobbs and Stephen Brown

Cover design: Bren Frisch
Illustrations: Susan Strawn Bailey and Gayle Ford

Text copyright 1997, Christopher Hobbs

Botanica Press is an imprint of Interweave Press

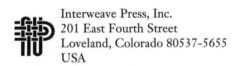 Interweave Press, Inc.
201 East Fourth Street
Loveland, Colorado 80537-5655
USA

Printed in the United States of America

Library of Congress Cataloging-in-Publication Data

Hobbs, Christopher, 1944-
    Saw palmetto: the herb for prostate health / by Christopher
Hobbs and Stephen Brown
        p.   cm.
    Includes bibliographical references and index
    ISBN 1-883010-46-2

First printing: 5M:1097:PP

Acknowledgments

A special thanks to Beth Baugh for help with every aspect of this project, from research and editing to personal encouragement. My gratitude also to Rick Mendosa for an incredible web site with good intentions (http://www.cruzio.com/~mendosa/sawpalm.html). Doree Pitkin provided her excellent editorial skills, and to all the people at Interweave Press who made this book a reality, my special appreciation.

CONTENTS

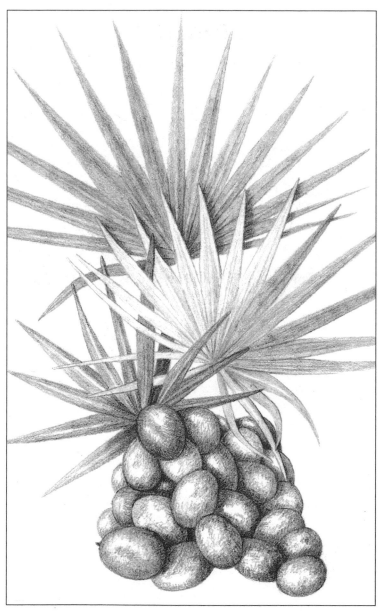

Saw Palmetto

INTRODUCTION

This book is written for every man over 50. This time of life ought to be one of the best, but almost half the men in this age group are troubled with urinary symptoms associated with enlarged prostate, a condition called benign prostatic hyperplasia (BPH). It is called benign because the enlargement is not cancerous; hyperplasia means increased growth. The symptoms of BPH include urinary urgency, frequent and uncomfortable urination both day and night, reduced urine flow, dribbling, and other annoying problems.

Maintaining prostate health and easing symptoms of an enlarged prostate are major challenges for older men, in part because the exact causes of the problem are not fully understood. In this book, you will find up-to-date information about BPH, discover the modern Western medical view of BPH, and learn ways to treat it.

You will also read about the alternative treatments for BPH that may be employed by herbalists or naturopaths. Natural systems of medicine, which include the use of healing herbs, diet, exercise, and relaxation techniques, can reduce and prevent symptoms associated with BPH. Such natural approaches are thousands of years old and used throughout the world to support and restore health; here they are explained in detail.

Extracts of the fruits of saw palmetto, a small palm that grows in the southeastern United States, have long been noted as effective to support prostate health. Research now shows that this safe, simple preparation may equal widely prescribed pharmaceutical preparations in treating BPH, without the side effects. Other herbs that contribute to prostate health also are reviewed in this book.

A Personal Story

Several years ago, my dad told me about some troublesome symptoms he was having: dizziness, nausea, and feeling disconnected. His usual nighttime trips to the bathroom disrupted his sleep, too. I asked him what he had been doing differently recently—Any new foods? A change in exercise? Increased stress? No, he replied.

Then Dad remembered that he had visited his doctor a month earlier, complaining of nighttime urination and daytime urinary discomfort. Dad's doctor, an affable fellow, checked Dad's prostate gland and found it was enlarged and probably contributing to the urinary symptoms. Dad went home with a prescription for a medication that's effective against BPH, but these other problems began about the same time.

Later I looked up the side effects of the drug Dad was taking, and every troubling symptom he described was listed. I recommended that he discontinue the drug and begin immediately to take an extract of saw palmetto fruit. In my clinic, I recommend this herbal remedy often to patients with prostate enlargement and uncomfortable urinary tract symptoms. It's safe and effective, and I thought it might help Dad.

After three weeks of taking the extract, Dad felt improved. After three or four months on the saw palmetto, he still had symptoms—a tough case, maybe. We increased his dose of herbal extract, and within another month, his symptoms began to decrease. After two months, they had completely disappeared! (I'm happy to say that now Dad sleeps through the night, which he feels is nearly a miracle. He has become a big fan of saw palmetto!)

A short time later, Dad returned to his doctor for a regular checkup. The doctor wanted to know if he was still getting up in the night, or if he had any less discomfort with urination. Dad replied, "Those symptoms are gone. I sleep fine through the night."

"Great," replied the doctor. "The prescription I gave you must have worked well!"

"Not at all," Dad answered. "In fact, I stopped taking it several months ago. My son recommended an herb, saw palmetto, and it seems to have done the job."

"Oh," said the doctor. "I'm taking that, too."

Treating benign prostatic hyperplasia is challenging because the gland and its functions are complex and not fully understood. It's helpful, then, to review the prostate's anatomy and actions with an eye to understanding as much as possible about this uniquely male structure.

Anatomy of the Prostate

The healthy prostate is a firm gland composed of both muscular and glandular tissue. Located beneath the male's urinary bladder, the prostate is about the size of a walnut and is shaped like a doughnut. It normally weighs about 20 grams, or just short of an ounce, and is essential to ejaculation.

The functions of the prostate gland and the urethra are closely related. The urethra is a tube that carries urine from the bladder through the "doughnut hole" of the prostate. As it passes through the prostate, the urethra is joined by the *vas deferens,* the tube that carries sperm from the testicles to the urethra, as well as many tiny ducts from the seminal vesicles. From that point onward, the urethra carries both urine and semen.

Usually the urethra carries urine from the bladder to the penis where it is ex-

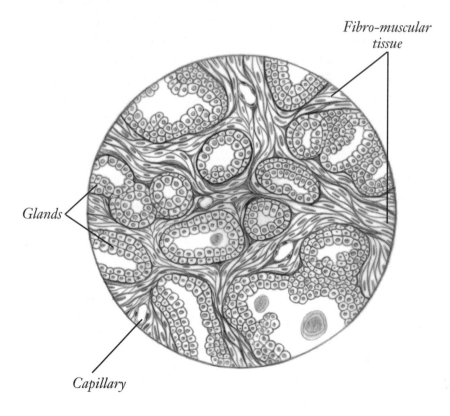

Fibro-muscular tissue

Glands

Capillary

Glandular tissue of the prostate, greatly magnified.

pelled; the prostate gland is quiet. During sexual activity, however, the prostate gland becomes active and the details of its structure are important.

Behind and on each side of the urethra as it passes through the prostate are areas of tissue called the central zone and the peripheral zone. The central zone, toward the top, contains irregular masses of secreting cells surrounded by thick fibromuscular tissue that forms a supporting latticework. The lower back and side portions, or the peripheral zone, contain smaller masses of secreting cells and fibromuscular tissues.

The forward portion of the gland is composed of fibromuscular tissue, including muscle that is continuous with the involuntary muscle sphincter of the bladder. This muscle keeps the bladder closed off prior to urination, and during sexual activity it seals the bladder to prevent urine from escaping into the urethra. Another part of this muscle forms the preprostatic sphincter, which prevents semen from flowing backwards into the bladder during ejaculation.

The bottom of the forward portion of the prostate contains muscle tissue that is continuous with the striated or voluntary sphincter below. This is the sphincter that one consciously relaxes when urinating.

During ejaculation, smooth muscles around the glandular part of the prostate expel the semen into the urethra and propel it out of the penis. The semen is composed of sperm in its nutritive plasma and secretions from the prostate, the seminal vesicles, and other glands. Prostate secretions make up about 25 percent of the semen's volume.

After ejaculation, the semen clots or thickens to protect the sperm from the hostile environment of the

vagina. After other sub-
stances modify the vaginal
environment to make it
friendlier to the sperm, enzymes from the prostate
liquefy the clot, freeing the
sperm to swim up through
the cervix into the uterus in
pursuit of a mature egg to
fertilize. In these ways the
prostate is essential to normal sexual activity.

A LOOK AT WHAT CAN GO WRONG

As men age, they are
quite likely to develop uri-
nary-tract symptoms that
can be attributed to benign
prostatic hyperplasia
(BPH). Autopsies show evidence of prostatic changes
in more than 40 percent of
men in their 50s and nearly
90 percent of men in their
80s (Berry 1984). More recent community-based
studies show prostate en-
largement among approxi-
mately 40 percent of men
in their 70s (Garraway
1991; Jacobsen 1995).

Not all men develop
symptoms from these
changes, however; nor is
there necessarily a correla-
tion between prostate size
and symptoms (Ohnishi et
al 1987). Although men
with enlarged prostates are
more likely to have symp-
toms, some men with en-
larged prostates have none,
while others with small
prostates have significant
symptoms. These facts indicate that a factor other than
mere overgrowth of the
gland often plays a part in
the symptoms blamed on
benign prostatic hyperplasia
(Shapiro 1995).

The first symptom men
usually notice when they're
developing an enlarged
prostate is decreased force
of the urine stream. Urination may be delayed or difficult to start or restart. Many
men experience a pressing
need to urinate, feeling
they're unable to wait. They
may find themselves need-
ing to urinate more often,
including several times dur-

A CAUTIONARY NOTE

A recent article in the journal *Medical Anthropology* provides a perspective on what is called the social construction of benign prostatic hypertrophy as a problematic disease (Mc-Dade 1996).

Studies show that men in various countries, including the United States, have similar age-related rates of BPH. Yet men in the United States are two to three times more likely to be diagnosed with BPH than men elsewhere. Treatment rates in the United States are much higher than in other countries, and prostatectomy rates have risen greatly since 1965. Treatment decisions are based primarily on the symptoms reported by the patient, despite the fact that symptoms don't necessarily indicate whether serious disease is present or not.

In other words, in the United States benign prostatic hypertrophy seems to be over-diagnosed and overtreated. Physicians' attitudes and economic desires and pharmaceutical companies' promotions have created a climate in which symptoms that are considered a normal part of aging in many parts of the world are imbued with ominous significance in the United States.

Of course, prostate symptoms should not be ignored, but one should take care that concerns about symptoms that may be part of the normal aging process don't lead to invasive treatment such as surgery, the risks and discomforts of which may be greater than the risks and discomfort from prostate enlargement.

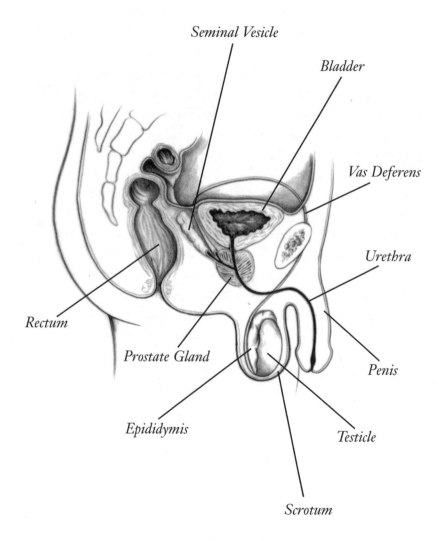

The male genitourinary tract.

ing the night, a condition called *nocturia*. When urination is completed, the bladder may not feel empty (and this is usually accurate), and annoying leaking and dribbling may occur. By the age of 55, 25 percent of men notice changes in their urine flow. By the age of 75, 50 percent of men notice a diminution of the force of the urine stream and greater than 90 percent of men in their 80s have some symptoms.

Origins of BPH

Benign prostatic hyperplasia is a noncancerous overgrowth of both the epithelial and fibromuscular cells of the prostate gland. This growth is controlled by a complex interaction of hormones and other factors secreted by the testicles, and by local tissue-growth factors secreted from cells in the prostate (Kyprianou 1996). When an overgrown prostate causes urinary difficulties, it is thought to be because nodular tissue in the transitional zone, and especially in the peri-urethral area, presses on the urethra as it passes through the prostate, obstructing the flow of urine.

There are substantial individual differences in the development of prostate overgrowth. The ratio of epithelial tissue to smooth muscle tissue in cases of BPH can vary from 1:3 to 4:1 (Price 1990).

Functional testes are required for BPH to develop, because testosterone, the major male hormone, and to a lesser extent estrogen, stimulate growth of normal prostate tissues. In the prostate, testosterone is converted to dihydrotestosterone (DHT) by an enzyme called 5α-reductase. DHT binds to androgen receptors in the prostate and stimulates cell proliferation.

High levels of DHT exist in normal prostate tissue. Testosterone levels, however, decline as men age, the same time that the prostate becomes enlarged. Animal studies show that prostate tissue continues to grow even when the testosterone-producing cells of the testes are destroyed. So it may well be that another unidentified substance secreted by the testes stimulates prostate-tissue growth. A number of studies have shown that nontestosterone factors secreted by the testes stimulate prostate-tissue growth (Lee 1995).

Contributing Factors to BPH

The list of factors that contribute to BPH remains incomplete, and some of the suspected causes are unproven. Some of the possibilities at present include the following:

- Inactivity reduces blood flow to the prostate and interferes with proper digestion and removal of wastes. Inactivity may also decrease immune-system function.

- A diet that is high in fat and sugar but low in fiber provides poor nutrition and elimination.

- Stress inhibits blood flow, suppresses immune activity, and affects the balance of hormones.

- Psychological responses can make it difficult to initiate urination.

- Some pharmaceutical drugs can aggravate symptoms of prostate trouble, among them the antidepressants Effexor and Paxil, the antihypertensive Hylorel, and Demodex, a diuretic.

Other Causes of Symptoms

Benign prostatic hyperplasia is not the only condition that causes urinary difficulties. For this reason, it's important to get an accurate diagnosis when any physical change occurs.

Aging. Age-related changes in the bladder and sphincter muscles often contribute to symptoms blamed on BPH. The muscles of the bladder weaken from age and from such conditions as diabetes, which causes nerve degeneration and a lack of sensation. Less efficiency at pushing the urine through the urethra leaves some urine in the bladder. In addition, the pushing of the bladder muscles against the urethra increases their mass. Over time, the muscles are replaced by less elastic connective tissue that further weakens the bladder. Imbalances in the muscle tissue lead to decreased ability to relax the urethral sphincter to allow free flow of urine. When the urethra is constricted by the enlarged prostate, symptoms are compounded.

Prostodynia. Some cases diagnosed as prostatitis manifest primarily as pain, especially in the perineum, without inflammation of the prostate. Such cases would better be classified as prostodynia—pain from the prostate—that does not involve inflammation. There may be some value in viewing chronic prostate pain as a chronic pain syndrome and taking a more multidisciplinary approach to its treatement (Egan 1997).

Prostatitis is an inflammation of the prostate tissue, and its symptoms are similar to those of BPH. The inflammation can have infectious or noninfectious origins and can be acute or chronic. Prostatitis, more common among young men, may occur at any age and includes urinary obstruction with pain, frequency and urgency, sexual symptoms like pain on ejaculation and impotence, and pain in the perineum, testicles, penis, and lower abdomen. Lower back pain is possible as well, but is more common in BPH.

Prostatitis is usually the result of infection. Its symptoms, which are identical to those of prostatism, are generally treated with antibiotics, sitz baths, bed rest, and fluids. Nonetheless, prostatitis, especially the chronic condition, has provoked one urologist to remark, "The management of prostatitis remains a frustrating problem for the clinical urologist. The various disease processes are poorly understood, the clinical presentation is extremely variable, the definitive diagnosis is difficult, and treatment is dismal" (Nickel 1995). Although half of all men experience symptoms of prostatitis at some time in their lives, in more than 90 percent of cases the cause is unknown (Krieger 1996).

Acute bacterial prostatitis is the most easily diagnosed and treated type, because the offending bacteria can frequently be cultured from urine or prostatic secretions. Treatment with an appropriate antibiotic follows. Bacterial prostatitis can become chronic because relapse after treatment is common.

Unfortunately, many cases of prostatitis have no discernible bacterial origin. Many physicians prescribe antibiotics on the presumption that undetected bacteria are causing the trouble, arousing concern that the overuse of antibiotics may strengthen drug-resistant microorganisms and eventually increase the incidence of chronic prostatitis.

Nonbacterial causes of inflammation include reflux or backflow of urine into the prostatic ducts (Persson 1996). Prostatitis symptoms can also arise from abnormal contractions of the sphincter muscles during urination, narrowing or obstructions that interfere with urine flow, and abnormalities in bladder-muscle activity (Kaplan 1997).

Psychological factors may often play an important role in chronic prostatitis. Depression and psychosocial distress are common among chronic prostatitis patients (Berghuis 1996). These conditions might lead to an immune suppression that encourages chronic infection. There are undoubtedly both cause-and-effect aspects of psychological difficulties associated with the symptoms of chronic prostatitis.

BPH and Prostatitis

At times prostatitis and BPH may coexist. There is no proven link between the two, but inflammation is thought to play a part in the etiology of many cases of BPH. Like BPH, prostatitis is very common, affecting half of all men. In a Croatian study, the incidence of prostatitis in BPH patients was over 90 percent, and over 60 percent showed evidence of bacterial prostatitis (Bedalov 1994). In one study, twenty of sixty-four samples of BPH tissue showed signs of immune-cell activity and nine of those tested positive for *Chlamydia*, a specialized bacteria that causes the most common sexually transmitted disease (Corradi 1996).

Prostatitis may be among the factors that push BPH to the clinically troublesome stage (Isaacs 1994). Although it may not *cause* BPH, prostatitis is often a part of the picture. Many believe, however, that the association between prostatitis and prostate cancer is better understood.

PROSTATE CANCER

The symptoms associated with BPH can also be caused by prostatic cancer. While men with BPH do not have a higher incidence of prostate cancer than others (Coley 1997), the relatively high rate of prostate cancer in the general population makes accurate diagnosis of symptoms essential. Over 40,000 men die of prostate cancer each year, making it the second leading cause of cancer death for American men (Wingo 1995). One in five men has a *lifetime* probability of being diagnosed with prostate cancer.

Although all the causative factors of prostate cancer have not been identified, it is likely that diet, exercise, and exposure to environmental toxins like herbicides play a role (Hubbard et al 1994). At least one-third of these cancers might be avoided if men made healthy dietary changes such as eliminating red meat and most animal fat from the diet and increasing their intake of fruits and vegetables (Wil-

lett 1995). A review study of existing data on prostate-cancer patients showed that for those with metastatic prostate cancer (stage D2), there is a statistically significant association between a healthy diet and survival with improved quality of life (Carter et al 1993).

Also diet-related is the fact that Asian men have distinctly lower prostate cancer rates than American men. The Japanese eat less animal fat and more vegetables and legumes such as tofu. For similar reasons, prostate cancer is almost nonexistent among Chinese men living in China. Japanese and Chinese men who come to the United States and begin eating a standard American diet, however, show a much higher incidence of the disease.

CHAPTER 1

EVALUATING
PROSTATE HEALTH

E xamination of the prostate should be part of the annual check-up of every man over 40. Early detection of problems is a positive factor in healing.

SYMPTOM QUESTIONNAIRES

Needing a questionnaire that accurately evaluates the severity of benign prostatic hyperplasia symptoms, the American Urological Association worked with a group of experts to develop the *AUA Symptom Score Index*. The questions concern the frequency of urination, urgency, steadiness of urine flow, and feelings of bladder fullness after urination. The patient rates his symptoms on a scale of 0 (not at all) to 5 (always). The answers to the questions help the health-care practitioner decide whether intervention is necessary. The questionnaire, which has been thoroughly tested for reliability and validity, provides a numerical representation of the severity of an individual's symptoms.

The World Health Organization also has adopted a questionnaire, the International Prostate Symptom Score. From the answers, a numerical score rates the difficulty of the patient's symptoms. Neither index is meant to be used as a screening test or sole diagnostic method, but both are useful as a follow-up for evaluating treatment outcomes.

THE DIGITAL RECTAL EXAMINATION

The digital rectal examination of the prostate is the most common way to check the health of the gland. Although this examination yields subjective and not highly specific or sensitive results, it does provide a general indication of prostate health.

The digital rectal examination should be used in conjunction with other tests to determine the health of the prostate. The healthy prostate is soft and smooth. One that is hard, nodular, or asymmetrical may warrant biopsy, even if other tests are negative. Biopsy sometimes detects cancers missed by other tests.

THE PROSTATE-SPECIFIC ANTIGEN TEST

The prostate-specific antigen test (PSA test), an early-detection blood test for prostate cancer, is typically used along with digital rectal examination and transrectal ultrasonography (an image made with ultrasound) in the diagnosis of prostate cancer.

Anyone being evaluated for symptoms of prostatism will be faced with the decision of whether to take a PSA test. Prostate-specific antigen, the substance detected by the test, is normally produced in quantity only in the prostate, hence its designation as prostate-specific. Prostate cancer often creates a rise in the level of this antigen in the blood. Benign prostatic hyperplasia also leads to an increase in the antigen, though not to the extent that cancer does (Stamey 1987). Easy access to PSA testing has resulted in the early detection, and thus early treatment, of many cases of prostate cancer.

THE PSA TEST CONTROVERSY

PSA testing is seriously debated in medical circles. National organizations disagree about its use. Currently the National Cancer Institute does not endorse mass PSA screening for prostate cancer. While the American Cancer Society and the American Urological Association support screening beginning at age 50, the American College of Physicians recommends against it (Sox 1997).

Controversy about the PSA test is based on its drawbacks. First, it may not help to save the lives of men with prostate cancer. In addition, PSA sensitivity and specificity are not high enough to eliminate uncertainty when interpreting the test.

Part of the problem lies in the fact that a number of benign situations can raise PSA levels. Two-thirds of men with a PSA value greater than 4, the usual cut-off value, turn out not to have cancer. PSA levels are often elevated by benign prostatic hyperplasia, prostatitis, and other non-cancerous conditions. Even a digital rectal exam can raise blood levels of PSA. For these reasons, the PSA test's sensitivity and specificity should be improved.

A medical test's sensitivity refers to its accuracy in detecting the disease for which it is used. A test that detects present illness a high percentage of the time is said to have a high sensitivity; one that often misses the present illness, giving a false-negative result, has a low sensitivity. The more false negative results given by a test, the lower the sensitivity, and the fewer the false negatives, the higher the sensitivity.

Because one's PSA is not always elevated, or elevated to a particular warning level, in the presence of prostate cancer, it's not unusual for the PSA test to give a normal reading when cancer is present, giving a *false-negative* reading. While the PSA test has a fairly high sensitivity, it is not ideal. The positive-predictive value, which is the percentage of men who test positive and have the disease, is less than 25 percent (Coley 1997).

A medical test's specificity measures how often a *positive* test result provides an accurate diagnosis of the disease. In other words, it takes into consideration how often the test gives positive results when the patient has cancer; or *false positives*, when the patient doesn't have cancer. Studies of PSA test's specificity have demonstrated varying results. One revealed a specificity of about 60 percent (Catalona 1991). A more re-cent prospective study showed a specificity of over 90 percent, with only 96 of 1,098 men who remained free of cancer having a false-positive result (Gann 1995).

Screening with the PSA test may do more harm than good when a false-positive result leads to unnecessary treatment for cancer. As many as 40 percent of men treated for prostate cancer have short-term incontinence; for some, the problem lasts longer. As many as 90 percent become sexually inactive. There is no strong evidence that PSA screening and treatment of prostate cancer decreases the number of deaths or incidents of disease associated with the cancer. Many men who would have gone through life without the likelihood of developing prostate cancer now must live with the fears and concern generated by a false-positive test.

Despite its uncertainties, the PSA test can detect

many prostate cancers at an early and potentially treatable stage. Over 40 percent of men over fifty develop prostate cancer (McConnel 1994) but only 20 to 25 percent of them will ever develop clinically apparent cancer, and only one out of eight men diagnosed with prostate cancer die of it (McConnel 1994). A cost-effectiveness study has determined that a one-time PSA test and digital rectal exam would lengthen the life of the average man between the ages of 50 and 69 by two weeks. Men over 69 would gain, at best, only a few days (Coley 1997). These statistics, along with the side effects of cancer treatment, should be considered.

Improving the PSA Test

We hope the future offers tests that will detect cancer with greater sensitivity and specificity and distinguish cancers that are likely to become life-threatening from those that are unaggressive. We also need treatments for prostate cancer that are effective but do not produce drastic side effects (Garnick 1996).

Several refinements in PSA testing are under way. One seeks to determine the ratio of free to total PSA in the blood (Catalona 1995; Partin 1996). Much of the PSA in the blood is bound to other proteins, but some is free or unbound, and men with aggressive cancers have been found to have a higher proportion of bound PSA than men with slow-growing cancers. The ratio of free-to-total PSA may help determine if a cancer is likely to grow aggressively (Metter 1997; Carter 1997). It may also be helpful in distinguishing prostate cancer from benign prostatic hyperplasia (Van Cangh 1996), thus identifying men who can benefit from watchful waiting and helping to avoid unnecessary harmful treatments.

Another way to increase the sensitivity of PSA testing is to measure PSA velocity, or the change in the individual's PSA over time. The rate of change helps to distinguish benign prostatic hyperplasia from cancer (Carter 1992): an increase of more than 20 percent in one year arouses suspicion of cancer.

OTHER PROSTATE TESTS

Other tests sometimes used in conjunction with the PSA test are proving helpful in evaluating prostate health. Using DNA from biopsied specimens, researchers have been able to distinguish cancerous from noncancerous prostate tissue 100 percent of the time (Malins 1997). Work is now underway to determine if a protein called kallikrein, which is present in the blood of men known to have prostate cancer, may be helpful when used to identify cancers not detected by PSA (Tindall 1997).

In the future, one hopes, new tests will allow a higher degree of certainty in diagnosing prostate conditions and their severity. At present, however, prostate testing remains insufficient.

CHAPTER 2

SAW PALMETTO AND OTHER HERBS FOR MEN

Herbs have been used as medicine throughout human history, and today they are the main source of medicine for most of the world's population. In the recent past of the Western world, many relied upon homemade herbal medicine to treat injuries, illnesses, and discomforts because doctors, if available, were poorly trained and employed scientific theories that were unproved or unfounded. Beginning about 120 years ago, however, the strictly scientific view of medicine began to gain ground and eventually displaced herbal medicines.

Nearly every culture has kept records of helpful plants, and the history of numerous medicinal herbs reaches back to the beginning of the written word. Many cultures have maintained oral records, and those relying on pictorial history have often painstakingly drawn out the details of helpful herbs and their uses. Although cultures have differed in their preferred uses of particular herbs, in many cases the usefulness of any one herb is the same in cultures around the world.

The gentle effectiveness of herbs, along with their reduced side effects and moderate cost, makes using them medicinally an attractive option in today's world. As interest in herbs increases, herbs and herbal products become more widely available.

USING HERBS SAFELY

As a general rule, to moderate potential individual reactions, any herbal treatment program ought to begin with a partial dose and work up to a full dose. Different herbs should be taken differently, according to their actions and the patient's condition.

Herbal remedies with specific actions, such as goldenseal and echinacea, are usually taken only when needed. After a course of treatment of two or three weeks for a particular condition, these remedies should be discontinued.

Some herbs are best taken in cycles, perhaps taken for ten days, discontinued for three days, and

taken for ten days again. This regimen gives the body time to rest and maintains the herb's maximum effectiveness. Tonic herbs, such as astragalus, reishi, and shiitake, can be taken for long periods of time, up to a year or more.

INDIVIDUAL CONSTITUTION

While herbs can be helpful for many conditions, to use them to their full potential it is important to consider one's individual constitution as well as the nature or "energetics" of the herb. A person who has a "cold" constitution benefits from herbs that warm the body by increasing metabolism or blood flow or tonic herbs that support and nourish the tissues. If one's constitution or present condition is hot, heat-clearing herbs (anti-inflammatories) are recommended.

Indicators of a cold or deficient constitution

include symptoms such as fatigue, depression, insomnia, and anxiety. Persons with a cold constitution tend to feel cold often, even if it isn't chilly, and seek out warm places. For them, tonic herbs such as ginseng, eleuthero, astragalus, reishi, and shiitake are advised. These tonics supply minerals and polysaccharides that support and nourish body processes and can help strengthen the immune system, hormonal system, and nervous system. For someone with a deficiency condition, taking tonifying herbs will generally expedite the healing process.

Someone with a hot, or excess, constitution may have symptoms such as infections, headaches, skin rashes, arthritis, and other inflammatory disorders. If an infection is mild but continues for weeks or months, the person may have a deficient immune system. This type of "pathogenic" (disease-causing)

heat is called "false heat," and mild antibacterial or heat-clearing herbs such as echinacea or yellow dock can help reduce it by fighting the infection and strengthening the immune system.

A person who is truly a hot and excess type tends to be robust. Such people will have a full pulse, and any infection they suffer is likely to be strong with fever; practitioners often see a thick, yellow coating on the tongue (no coating or slight coating occurs with false-heat conditions). True excess types tend to have strong hereditary constitutions and eat lots of red meat and fats; they often develop heart disease. Herbs that benefit heat conditions are cooling, such as goldenseal, coptis, barberry, woad (isatis), or andrographis. For conditions of both excess and deficiency, it is wise to seek the aid of a practitioner of Traditional Chinese Medicine or

BPH AND TRADITIONAL CHINESE MEDICINE

In China, researchers have studied the effects of two common treatment strategies according to the ancient system of healing, Traditional Chinese Medicine (TCM). The first is "Invigorating Blood and Resolving Masses," and the second is "Tonifying the Kidneys". Western medicine believes that blood circulation plays an important role in benign prostatic hypertrophy, and the same approach is considered relevant in TCM (Xie et al 1994).

In Chinese medicine, the "Kidney" is a metaphor for the working of hormones and neurotransmitters and the potential of the body's cells to produce energy. These functions can be damaged by long-term stress. In TCM, kidney tonics are used to help correct this problem, and they include "adaptogen" herbs from Western herbalism.

The best-studied adaptogens are eleuthero, rehmannia, ligustrum, American ginseng, and ashwaganda, all of which are widely available. A practitioner of TCM can complete a personal diagnosis and treatment plan using traditional guidelines and combining TCM with modern Western, nutritional, herbal, and drug treatments to help relieve symptoms. TCM treatments address underlying "constitutional" metabolic imbalances. Each form of medicine increases the effectiveness of the other.

herbalist trained in natural or constitutional medicine to prescribe these herbs appropriately.

Conditions of excess and deficiency can accompany prostate inflammation and benign prostatic hyperplasia. While saw palmetto can be useful in relieving inflammation, it is more effective when combined with other herbs that help balance the underlying constitutional condition. Further, combining herb intake with healthy habits and stress-release methods will promote further healing and lead to greater overall health and enjoyment of life.

SAW PALMETTO AND HOW TO USE IT

Saw palmetto is a small palm, *Serenoa repens*, that is native to the coastal regions of the southeastern United States. It belongs to the botanical family Arecaccae and is related to the true palmettos from the genus *Sabal*. Botanists formerly called saw palmetto *Sabal serrulata*. Its natural habitat is pinelands, coastal dunes, and sand hills from Charleston, South Carolina, south through Florida and west to Louisiana.

Highly variable in its growth habits, saw palmetto is a hardy plant. The stems sometimes branch and can grow flat to the ground or become buried. Other times the stem grows upright to twelve to twenty feet. Three to seven fan-shaped leaves develop from the stem each year. The leaves endure for more than a year, giving the plant the typical palm appearance with new leaves growing above the older, dying leaves and old leaf scars. Judging by the leaf scars and the length of growing stems, it has been estimated that some older plants are 500 to 700 years old.

A cluster of white flowers grows in the spring; the flowers are an important source of nectar and pollen for bees and other pollinating insects. Clusters of green fleshy fruits, each surrounding a stone that contains a single seed, develop by May or June. Technically described as a drupe, the fruit ripens through the summer, becoming bluish-black in the fall, by which time many have fallen off or been eaten by animals and insects.

Saw palmetto provides important habitat and a source of food for wildlife. Black bears are said to become sleek and healthy eating the berries and the starchy growing ends of the stems. Being resistant to insects, drought, and fire, and requiring no fertilizer, saw palmetto is a popular choice for landscaping in its native areas.

History of Use

It's reported that Native American Indians consumed fresh or dried saw palmetto berries as a tonic food. They also used tannin from saw palmetto stems to cure hides and the leaves and branches to make brooms, hats, and baskets.

The medical world took interest in the herb in the late 1800s when farmers observed that animals appeared exceptionally healthy after consuming saw palmetto fruits. Practitioners began decocting saw palmetto, word of its benefits spread, and many articles about its effects appeared. Believed to have an alterative, health-promoting action on the genitourinary tract and recommended for enlarged prostate in elderly men, the herb was also credited with tonifying the mucous membranes of the bladder and urethra (*U.S. Dispensatory*, 1877).

Active around the turn of the century, Eclectic physicians used herbs almost exclusively in their practices. Dr. I. J. M. Goss, an Eclectic physician, stated that he "had been induced to use the remedy [saw palmetto] and considered it satisfacto-ry" (*Medical Brief* 1877). In the Felter-Lloyd revision (1898) of the well-known *King's American Dispensatory*, the actions and uses of saw palmetto are summarized.

Actions: Nutritive tonic; expectorant (clears mucus), controls irritation of mucous membranes

Uses: Irritable coughs, chronic bronchial coughs, whooping cough, acute and chronic laryngitis, asthma. Digestive tonic, improving appetite, digestion, and assimilation. Its most important effect is on the genitourinary tracts of both sexes; it strengthens and enlarges wasted organs such as the breasts, ovaries, and testicles, but reduces the hypertrophied prostate [Felter and Lloyd explained this inconsistency by defining saw palmetto as an amphoteric; that is, it *normalized* the size and function of organs.] It restores sexual activity after exhaustive excesses; long-continued use slowly and

surely causes breast enlargement.

In one regard, Felter and Lloyd anticipated the most important modern use of saw palmetto by nearly a century. Calling it "the old man's friend," they said the herb relieves many annoyances commonly attributed to enlarged prostate. The authors noted that its specific indications and uses include prostatic irritation, painful urination, and dribbling of urine, particularly in the aged.

F. J. Petersens's *Materia Medica and Clinical Therapeutics* of 1905 states, "We think of [saw palmetto] in enlarged prostate, atrophy of the testes or uterus, and all prostatic troubles. . . . [Saw palmetto] has a direct influence upon the glands of the reproductive system, as mammae, ovaries, prostate, testes, etc., increasing their functional activity and tending to bring about normal action and size."

By the early 1920s, saw palmetto was considered one of the most important remedies used in the South (Lloyd 1921). Saw palmetto was official in the *U.S. Pharmacopoeia* from 1900 to 1916 and in the *National Formulary* from 1925 to 1942.

USING SAW PALMETTO

If you happen to live in eastern Florida or other parts of the southeastern United States where saw palmetto grows abundantly, you can pick and dry your own fruit. The whole dried fruits can also be purchased from many herb shops or herb suppliers. Grind them into powder in a blender or coffee grinder and pack them into 00-size capsules to avoid the taste, which some find unpleasant. Five grams of the fruit will fill ten capsules, the minimum daily therapeutic dose. If you don't find the smell or taste objectionable, sprinkle the fruit powder on cereal or add it to soups, stews, or other foods. Those without access to the whole fruit can choose from an amazing array of commercial products in every form: liquid tinctures, capsules, tablets, and teas. All contain the healing components of the saw palmetto fruit.

Extracts

Because of the inconvenience of preparing saw palmetto fruit and taking five to ten capsules daily, manufacturers extract what they believe to be the medicinal constituents of saw palmetto, leaving the other parts of the fruit behind. The extract becomes part of saw palmetto tinctures, tablets, capsules, and teas. Although many believe in the efficacy of such products, German chemists and pharmacologists believe that the whole plant contains a complex mixture of compounds that work together to produce a much more balanced and beneficial effect than that of highly purified, standardized extract. More research may give consumers more information to use when selecting products that contain saw palmetto.

When considering what kind of commercial product of saw palmetto to buy, there are some important factors to keep in mind. Three solvents are used to extract the herb's fatty-acid fraction, which is believed to be of medicinal benefit: industrial solvents such as hexane, grain alcohol, and liquefied carbon dioxide. We recommend avoiding products extracted with hexane or other industrial solvents, although they are often cheaper than others. Why risk adding even minute amounts of these chemicals to the body or environment when excellent alternatives are available?

Products extracted by grinding the dried fruits in ethanol (grain alcohol) contain some fatty acids

A LESSON IN STANDARDIZATION

Standardization does not always increase the effectiveness of an herb, as we've learned from studies of St. John's wort. Several years ago, manufacturers sold extracts standardized to higher levels of hypericin than exist in the herb, believing that hypericin contributes most to the activity of the herb. As time went on, studies and reports revealed that whole-plant extracts containing all the herb's compounds are more effective than standardized extracts.

This serves to warn that highly purified extracts of saw palmetto, standardized to fatty acids or sterols, can be effective, but the whole fruits eaten with food or placed in capsules should be considered effective as well.

and sterols. Little research has been done on the use of these extracts. They may be effective, but we need more information to determine how they compare to the whole fruit or the liquid carbon dioxide extracts.

The third, and probably most effective extraction method, is hypercritical carbon dioxide. In this process, carbon dioxide gas is frozen and pressurized to turn it into a liquid. This liquid is then used as a solvent to extract the fatty acids and sterols from saw palmetto fruits. Then the temperature of the carbon dioxide is increased until it returns to the gaseous state and evaporates, leaving behind the plant constituents. The beauty of this process is that the delicate fatty acids, which easily become rancid when exposed to heat and oxygen, are preserved in their original, undamaged state.

Whole fruits and standardized extracts are readily available through the mail and in supermarkets, drug stores, and natural products stores. Buying from the last supports organic foods and a variety of natural products. The most informed salespeople can be found in these stores as well, making it more likely that your questions about herbs will be answered accurately; those who work in drug stores and supermarkets typically know little or nothing about herbs.

Commercial extracts are not all of the same quality, although their labels may contain similar information. Many products claim to be standardized to 85 to 95 percent fatty acids and biologically active sterol compounds. Many manufacturers add olive oil or other oils as carriers. The cost of saw palmetto products varies widely, from 12 to 60 cents per capsule, depending on where you buy them (Mendosa 1997).

CULTIVATING SAW PALMETTO

The current demand for saw palmetto berries tops 20 million pounds a year, requiring about 175,000 acres of trees, and the market may grow by 10 percent per year. The trees are not difficult to cultivate; they resist drought, insects, and fire, and require no fertilizer. Saw palmetto berries have been harvested commercially for nearly a century, with crops destined primarily for the European herbal market. This direction changed dramatically in 1995, when a relaxed regulatory climate in the United States spurred interest in marketing saw palmetto products to aging baby-boomers for prostate problems. That year's small crop, coupled with increased demand, drove the price of saw palmetto berries from 10 cents a pound to over $2, exciting Southern farmers, wildcrafters, and migrant workers.

Interest in cultivating saw palmetto for commercial production is growing. European entrepreneurs have purchased Southern farms to establish saw palmetto plantations, and American cattle ranchers and farmers have formed a saw palmetto growers' cooperative. Some ranchers have found that cultivating saw palmetto is a more profitable use of their land than raising cattle (Vachon 1996).

Although the cooperative will probably press for increases in the price of saw palmetto, it may also help make consistently higher quality berries available. The group plans to study the growth habits of the tree and assess the impact of intensive annual harvests on wildlife, reflecting an awareness of the importance of preserving this precious natural ecosystem. The impact on wildlife and the trees themselves of newer, high-yield management methods, such as burning the saw palmetto fields prior to harvest, is now unknown.

Proper Dose

Scant valid testing of saw palmetto makes it difficult to determine the exact dose of the dried fruit, but clinical and dietary use can guide such decisions. The best clinical information we have on the use of saw palmetto is from the Eclectic physicians, whose clinical experience recorded in journals and texts is considered a rich storehouse of information by today's herbalists. According to Felter and Lloyd (1898), the Eclectic dose of the strong extract was one to sixty drops, up to two droppersful, most appropriately two to three times a day before meals. Today's dose of saw palmetto extract is up to one teaspoon (five droppersful) of the liquid, two to three times daily.

Capsule dosages vary somewhat by manufacturer, but a typical recommendation is one capsule (160 milligrams) twice a day, morning and evening, for light or moderate discomfort, and two capsules twice a day for great discomfort. Some manufacturers recommend a treatment cycle of thirty days or longer, repeated as necessary.

Safety and Side Effects of Saw Palmetto

The side effects of taking saw palmetto for months or longer seem to be minimal. One European product, Permixon, lists only one side effect: "Occasionally, nausea may occur, especially when the product is taken on an empty stomach." Some individuals may find themselves allergic to the plant. Otherwise, saw palmetto, used as directed, is free of side effects.

SCIENTIFIC STUDIES OF SAW PALMETTO

Saw palmetto is a relatively new medicinal herb, so its use has not been documented over a great length of time. The Eclectic physicians employed the herb in the United States for several decades and saw palmetto has been harvested for the European market for about a century, but like other herbs, saw palmetto fell into disuse when modern pharmaceutical drugs became popular and widely available. Consequently, scientific studies, many of them European, give us the most reliable information about saw palmetto's effectiveness and safety.

Anyone suffering from the discomforts of disease asks two major questions about a potential treatment: Does it work?, and Is it safe? A related question is whether another treatment might be safer or more effective. The answers to these questions, particularly in regard to saw palmetto, are not always obvious or easy.

Study Design

Scientific studies are not easy reading, even for sci-entists. Yet the lay person who wants to know more about herbs often finds it necessary to peruse such studies to evaluate the herb, its uses, and its safety. Knowing a bit about the design of scientific studies helps in analyzing and evaluating the study's results.

Correct design is a major factor in the ultimate value of scientific studies. In general, poorly designed studies can yield information that is skewed or downright wrong, while well-designed studies can result in much more reliable data. The use of placebo and control groups, sufficient size of study, and length of study all contribute to validity.

Control Groups. Two or more groups of subjects are often involved in treatment tests. "Randomized" selection of subjects and their careful assignment to control or experimental groups prevents selection bias that interferes with objective assessment of the results. The experimental group receives the treatment being investigated, while the control group does not. Valid comparisons require that the subjects in each group be as similar as possible in all ways except for the treatment. For example, if obese people comprised the control group and thin people the experimental group, the comparison may not be valid because the groups may respond to the treatment differently.

Studies that do not include control groups are called open trials. In this type of study, all participants receive treatment. Open trials are valuable after randomized, controlled studies have indicated efficacy and safety of treatment, but as initial studies they are not appropriate.

Placebo Effect. The apparent effectiveness of any medicine, natural or synthetic, can be influenced by a placebo effect, a positive result caused by the patient's expectation of improvement with treatment, even if the treatment itself has no real effect. Some conditions seem to be particularly responsive to the placebo effect, and among these are the symptoms of benign prostatic hyperplasia (Schulze 1982; Meyhoff 1996; Nickel 1997).

Expectation can also influence the physician's or researcher's interpretation of particular treatment results. Knowing that a particular patient has received a treatment can lead to a substantial lack of objectivity in interpreting the results. Financial incentives can compromise objectivity as well, a possible outcome when research is funded by promoters of a drug under investigation. Attachment to a philosophical position, such as the promotion of "conventional" medical treatments over "alternative" therapies, or vice versa, can also interfere with objectivity. And all too often, negative studies—those that don't produce the hypothesized results—are not published.

Scientific studies are designed to neutralize the placebo effect, since any improvement it produces is unrelated to treatment. Because the placebo effect can originate with patient or supervisor, a "double-blind" design prevents either from knowing who receives treatment and who does not.

Study Size. The number of subjects in a study influences validity. If one flips a coin ten times, the chances of getting seven or eight of either heads or tails are quite high. With 1,000 flips, however, the likelihood of approaching half heads, half tails increases. Similarly, trials that involve larger numbers of subjects have a greater chance of statistical validity and are given more weight.

Length of Study. In general, long studies yield more high-quality information than short studies do. Long studies are likely to reveal the development of treatment effects, unwanted side effects, and long-term complications that are not apparent when treatment begins. Following patients for an extended period often yields valuable information.

Combining these factors creates randomized, double-blind, controlled studies. Such studies have greater legitimacy than studies that lack one or more factors.

Analyzing Study Results

The complex data produced by scientific studies, typically expressed numerically, require complex statistical analysis to produce accurate, useful conclusions. Reviewing methods of analysis is beyond the scope of this book, but it is important to understand some of the outcomes.

Statistically significant is a term sometimes used to

imply that a study has revealed information of great magnitude. However, the term really means that the reported difference between placebo and experimental group is probably not due to chance.

Consider a study that shows the drug being tested "significantly improves symptoms." If the study shows that the control group (which indicates placebo effect) improved by 40 percent, while the experimental group (which indicates treatment effect) improved by 45 percent, the treatment is only 5 percent better than no treatment at all. This result may be statistically significant, but it does not indicate that the experimental drug is a promising treatment.

Probability is another word easily misused in the discussion of scientific studies. The probability figure expresses the degree of likelihood that the study's results are due to chance alone. For instance, p value of .05 means that there are only five chances in 100 that the study's results are due to chance alone; a value of .01 means only one chance in 100. The lower the p value, the higher the validity of the experiment.

Reproducibility also affects the credibility of an experimental result. If others can follow the procedures of a given study and achieve the same results, the study is said to be reproducible and it gains greater credibility. Results that cannot be reproduced are considered highly suspect, if not bogus.

Peer review is the critical appraisal of an experiment by other knowledgeable scientists. It is typically used by scientific or academic journals. A panel of experts reviews each study proposed for publication to determine its validity and usefulness. Thus, studies that are published in "peer-reviewed" journals have greater import than those published in non-peer-reviewed publications, or those that have not been published at all.

The studies of saw palmetto's efficacy in the treatment of benign prostatic hyperplasia are subject to all these criteria and offer potential users a good deal of knowledge and guidance.

Studies of Treatments with Saw Palmetto

A number of studies have been done, both as open trials and double-blind studies (see Tables 2-1 and 2-2 at the end of this chapter). The quality of these studies varies considerably, but overall they indicate that saw palmetto is a safe and effective treatment for the symptoms of mild to moderate BPH. How effective saw palmetto is in comparison to other therapies remains unclear.

The course and manifestation of BPH vary greatly

from one patient to another. Over time, patients who initially present with the same severity of symptoms can evince great differences in the development of the disease on a tissue level and in symptoms; they can experience very different outcomes (Barry 1997). For this reason, studies have not yet given a clear picture of the disease and its course. So long as practitioners lack valid data, treatments for the problem will be varied in both substance and results.

While suggestive and interesting, many studies of saw palmetto's clinical efficacy are of questionable value because they do not include control groups. Many are open trials; that is, all patients are treated with the extract, and patients and researchers participate in evaluating the results. Several researchers have noted that BPH responds very well to the placebo effect; 40 to 60 percent of patients treated with placebo for BPH experience significant symptomatic improvement for up to two years (Schulze 1982; Lepor 1996; Nickel 1997). Open trials, even lengthy ones, may not yield useful information about the treatment of BPH with saw palmetto. This criticism is compounded by saw palmetto studies that are too short or lack objective data.

Yet several studies of saw palmetto have documented impressive results. A number of open trials have shown significant results in both objective and subjective parameters.

- One year-long trial found improvement of over 70 percent in symptoms such as hesitancy, weak or interrupted stream, and the feeling of having incomplete emptying of the bladder. After twelve months, 80 percent of patients were said to be symptom free. The number of urinations during the day decreased by 28.9 percent and at night by 37.8 percent. Residual urine—urine left in the bladder after urination—decreased from an average of 62.8 milliliters before the study to 12.3 milliliters after the study. Maximum flow rates increased from 11.0 ml/sec to 15.2 ml/sec stream (Romics, 1993).

- In another study of 435 patients, over 80 percent of the patients and their doctors described the overall results as either very good or good. Maximum urine flow was increased by 6.1 milliliters per second, and residual urine was decreased by 50 percent. The researcher reported a 73.3 percent response rate for nocturia, a 53.5 percent response rate for daytime frequency, and a 75.9 percent response in the sensation of incomplete emptying of the bladder (Bach 1996).

A few double-blind, placebo-controlled studies have been carried out. The majority of these have shown impressive results after treatment with saw palmetto extract, though the studies have been criticized for poor methodological quality. An often-quoted study of a commercial saw palmetto extract, Permixon, by Champault et al (1984) highlights some of the problems with these studies.

The study claims that nighttime urination decreased by 45.8 percent in the Permixon-treated group and only 15 percent in the placebo control group. Flow rates, which were unusually low at the beginning of the experiment, increased 50.5 percent in the

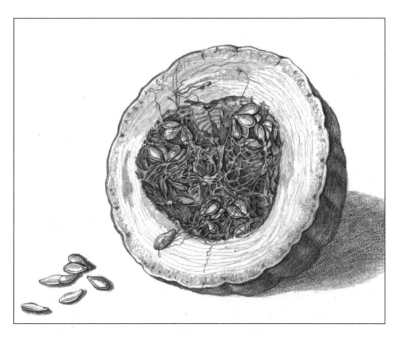

Pumpkin seed is believed by some to relieve symptoms of benign prostatic hyperplasia.

treated group and only 5 percent in the placebo group. Post-urination residual urine volumes decreased by 41.9 percent in the treated group and increased by 9.3 percent in the placebo group. Fourteen in the treatment group rated themselves "greatly improved" and 33 "improved".

This study has been criticized because the length of the experiment, only thirty days, was insufficient to evaluate the effects of treatment on BPH symptoms. Further, its rate of placebo response is very low compared to many other studies. A pronounced placebo effect is usually observed during treatment of benign prostatic hyperplasia, yet none of this placebo group rated themselves greatly improved, though 30 did rate themselves improved.

Although the criticisms of Champault's study are fair, on balance the data presented shows a fairly dramatic positive effect of saw palmetto extract on BPH. If the study can be replicated for a longer period, Champault's results can be confirmed or rejected.

Another placebo-controlled study of Permixon extract has given very different results (Reece-Smith, 1986). This twelve-week trial scored assessments by both patients and physicians of changes in BPH symptoms. As assessed by physicians, both experimental and control groups showed significant improvement. When the subjects reported their improvement, however, the control group (who did not receive treatment) reported improvement at a higher rate than the treatment group.

Several other double-blind, placebo-controlled studies compare various extracts of saw palmetto. Most show that treatment is more effective than placebo, by both objective and subjective measures. The likelihood of some de-

Table 2-1: Saw Palmetto Extract: Summary of Controlled Clinical Trials

Author, date	Extract & dose	Number of subjects	Study lengths	Treatment outcomes	Placebo outcomes
Descotes 1995	Permixon, 160 mg bid	176	1 mo.	PFR ↑ 29%; N ↓ 33%; P ↑ 11%	PFR ↑ 9%; N ↓ 18%; P ↓ 3%
Lobelenz 1992	Sabal extract, 100 mg tid	60	6 wks.	PFR–10%	PFR– 5%
Reece-Smith 1986	Permixon, 160 mg bid	70	12 wks.	PFR ↑ ~35%; N ↓ ~36%; P ↓ ~12%;	PFR ↑ ~35%; N ↓ ~ 36% P ↓ ~ 6%;
Tasca 1985	PA 109, 160 mg bid	30	2 mo.	PFR ↑ 26%; N ↓ 74%	PFR ↑ 5%; N ↓ 39%
Cukier 1985	Permixon, 160 mg bid	146	2-3 mo.	N ↓ 33%; P ↓ 20%	N ↓ 15%; P ↓ 1%
Champault 1984	Permixon, 160 mg bid	89	1 mo.	PFR ↑ 19%; N ↓ 46%	PFR ↑ 5%; N ↓ 15%
Emili 1983	Permixon 160 mg bid	30	1 mo.	PFR ↑ 33%; N ↓ 50%; P ↓ 32%	PFR ↑ 2%; N ↓ 13%; P ↓ 8%
Boccafoschi 1983	Permixon, 160 mg bid	22	2 mo.	PFR ↑ 43%; N ↓ 55%; P ↓ 29%	PFR ↑ 19%; N ↓ 32%; P ↓ 29%

Key: PFR = peak urinary flow rate; N = nocturia, frequency of nighttime urination; P = pollaciuria, frequency of daytime urination; PVR = post voiding residual urine; bid = twice a day; tid = three times a day.

gree of publisher's bias must be considered; advertisers often exert pressure on publishers to portray their products in a positive light.

Active Ingredients of Saw Palmetto Extract

The action of saw palmetto becomes more potent, simpler to implement, and more reliable when the herb is used in capsules, tablets, or liquid preparations. Extracts concentrate the active constituents and reduce the odor and taste of the whole fruits.

Extracts of *Serenoa repens* are composed mostly of fatty acids of varying chain lengths, with a small percentage of sterol compounds (Stenger 1982). The fatty-acid makeup of a hypercritical CO_2 extract is shown in Table 2-2, page 53 (Neiderprum 1994). Other analyses have demonstrated similar components in saw palmetto preparations. These extracts are called liposterol or lipophilic extracts because they contain fat-soluble compounds from the fruit. Saw palmetto also contains small amounts of polysaccharides and long-chain alcohols called polyprenols. Other secondary constituents include steroids (Stenger 1982), diterpenes, triterpenes, sesqueterpene, and alcohols.

Saw Palmetto Mechanisms

Because BPH symptoms often ease after patients take preparations of saw palmetto, many researchers have sought to isolate the herb's mechanism of action. Learning *how* and *why* saw palmetto works in the human body may allow the design of more effective extracts and make this herb available to millions of men worldwide.

Documented clinical work by trained and experienced herbalists, naturopaths, and physicians reports saw palmetto's effectiveness, helps to determine proper dose range, and describes how saw palmetto works within a total natural medicine program that includes diet and exercise. Overall, this body of work holds that saw palmetto extract contains an effective mechanism, but it does not address what that mechanism might be. Scientific studies have explored various possibilities, but the results are unclear.

β-**Sitosterol.** In one double-blind, placebo-controlled trial, 200 symptomatic BPH patients were given either twenty milligrams of β-sitosterol, a constituent of saw palmetto, or placebo three times a day (Berges et al 1995). The control group improved in peak urine flow and had decreased mean residual urinary retention volume, compared with the placebo group. Because β-sitosterol is available in many herbs and foods, saw

palmetto is not essential to obtain it.

Hormonal Studies of BPH

Studies of saw palmetto extract's ability to change the actions of hormones affecting the development of benign prostatic hyperplasia are similarly contradictory and unclear. Several possible ways that the herb may interfere with the hormones' actions on the prostate have been explored.

DHT. Dihydrotestosterone (DHT) stimulates growth of prostate tissue in both normal and hyperplastic prostate glands. It is formed from testosterone by the enzyme 5α-reductase, and those born with defects in the enzyme do not have normal growth of prostate tissue and never develop benign prostatic hyperplasia. Chemically interfering with the formation or action of DHT prevents and even to some extent reverses benign prostatic hyperplasia. These studies indicate that saw palmetto's *major* action cannot now be identified as the inhibition of 5α-reductase, though it is possible. The fatty acid environment in the prostate may change when saw palmetto is consumed over a period of time, thus decreasing enzyme activity, but more research is needed to confirm this theory. The fatty acids found in saw palmetto may also mediate clinical results in ways that are not yet understood.

Receptors. DHT must bind to prostate-cell receptors to stimulate growth. Some experiments have sought to determine if saw palmetto extracts interfere with binding. Several studies in the 1980s indicated that saw palmetto extracts

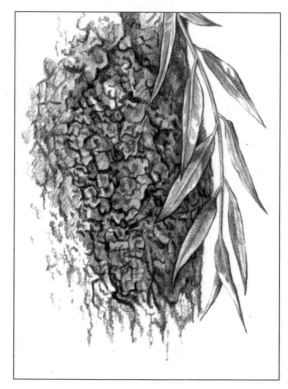

Preparations of willow (bark and leaf shown here) may relieve the inflammation of BPH.

Table 2-2: Saw Palmetto Extract: Summary of Open Uncontrolled Studies

Author, date	Extract & dose	Number of subjects	Study length	Objective outcomes	Subjective outcomes
Bach 1996	Sabal extract IDS 89, 160 mg bid	435	3 yrs.	PFR ↑ 46%; N ↓ 73%; P ↓ 54%; PVR ↓ 50%	Good or very good in 80%
Schneider 1995	Strogen Forte[1], 2 capsules per day	2,080	12 wks.	PFR ↑ 39%; N ↓ 49%; P ↓ 25%; PVR ↓ 42%;	Improvement in 85%
Braeckman 1994	Serenoa extract, 160 mg bid	505	3 mo.	PFR ↑ 25%; PVR ↓ 20%	Effective in 88%
Romics 1993	Strogen Forte 2 capsules per day	42	12 mo.	PFR ↑ 40%; N ↓ 38%; P ↓ 29%; PVR ↓ 79%	No symptoms in 80%
Vahlensieck 1993	Sabal extract, 160 mg bid	1,334	12 wks.	N ↓ 54%; P ↓ 37%; PVR ↓ 50%	Good to excellent in > 80%

Key: PFR = peak urinary flow rate; N = nocturia, frequency of nighttime urination; P = pollaciuria, frequency of daytime urination; PVR = post voiding residual urine

[1] Strogen Forte contains *Urtica* extract and *Sabal serrulata* extract.

interfered with this process, but more recent studies generally find that these effects are very limited or nonexistent.

Estrogen. The female hormone estrogen, made in small amounts in men's bodies, may influence prostate growth. Like DHT, it stimulates cells after binding at special receptor sites. One study (DiSilverio, 1992) found that saw palmetto extract decreases the number of receptor sites available for estrogen binding, thus limiting the action of the hormone.

Prolactin. This is another hormone that may stimulate prostate growth. Some research indicates that saw palmetto extract blocks prolactin receptors (Vacher 1995), although the study was done on rat prostate cells.

Inflammatory hormones. Saw palmetto may exert anti-inflammatory or antiedematous (anti-

swelling) actions on prostate tissues by inhibiting enzymes that produce prostaglandins and other inflammatory compounds from fatty acids (Tarayre 1983). One group of researchers (Hiermann et al 1989) demonstrated that the sterol and flavonoid components of saw palmetto extracts are not responsible for the anti-inflammatory effects.

Commission E Monograph

Commission E is a group of scientists, doctors, herbalists, regulators, and company representatives sponsored by the German government. The group reviews the world's literature on herbal medicines and writes guidelines on how the herbs can be used, including information about safety, side effects, dose, and uses. Commission E has published the following information about the saw palmetto berry.

Constituents: Saw palmetto berry consists of the ripe, dried fruit of *Serenoa repens* as well as its preparations in effective dosage. The drug contains fatty oil with phystosterols and polysaccharides.

Uses: Urination problems in benign prostatic hyperplasia, stages 1 and 2.

Contraindications: None known.

Side Effects: In rare cases, stomach problems.

Interactions with Other Drugs: None known.

Dosage: Daily: 1 to 2 grams berry or 320 milligrams lipophilic ingredients extracted with lipophilic solvents (hexane or ethanol, 90 percent by volume; or equivalent preparations.

Action: Antiandrogenic, antiexudative

Caution: This medication relieves only the diffi-

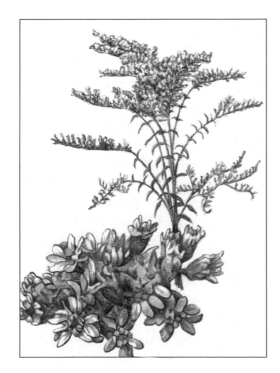

Teas and tinctures of golden-rod are said to increase blood circulation to the prostate.

culties associated with an enlarged prostate without reducing the enlargement. Please consult a physician at regular intervals.

OTHER MEN'S HERBS

Several other herbs have a history of use for easing the symptoms of benign prostatic hyperplasia. Only two, however, have consistently shown promise in this regard. See Table 2-3 for information about the herbs that have been examined for this purpose.

Urtica dioica (Stinging Nettle)

Nettle root—the roots and rhizomes (underground stems) of *Urtica dioica* and *Urtica urens*—is a popular herbal remedy for prostate enlargement with accompanying urinary symptoms. The herb, including leaves and stems, is highly regarded for treatment of urinary problems and as a nutritive tonic. Nettle contains high concentrations of bio-available minerals, especially iron, zinc, and magnesium. In Europe the extract is available in many formulations, often combined with saw palmetto, pygeum, and pumpkin-seed extracts. A small number of human clinical studies have been performed, but as with saw palmetto, only a few were controlled. Even then, the number of volunteers and the length of the studies make the results inconclusive from the standpoint of modern medicine.

Recent research has shown promising results in the treatment of BPH with nettle extract. In one study, cells from a sample of enlarged prostate tissue were exposed to the steroidal components of nettle root extract (Hirano 1994). The enzyme activity of the cells was inhibited, suggesting that nettle root extract may suppress the growth of prostate cells. Another study (Schmidt 1983) has shown

Table 2-3. Review of Men's Herbs for the Prostate

Herb	Source	Dose	Study Findings	Uses
Saw palmetto	Powdered fruits, ethanolic extracts, powdered extracts	160 mg/day	Credible double-blind studies	Reduces prostate swelling, pain; improves urine flow
Flower pollen	*Standardized powdered extract	2 tablets, 3 x daily of Cernilton	A few double-blind studies	Reduces swelling, improves urine flow
Pygeum	Standardized powdered extract	—	Some credible studies	Reduces prostate swelling, pain, improves urine flow
Nettle root	Tea, liquid and standardized powdered extracts	2-4 grams of powdered extract; 1 tsp. of the ethanolic tincture, 2-3 times daily	Only a few studies	Reduces prostate swelling, pain; improves urine flow
Pumpkin seed extract	Oil or powders standardized to fatty acids; whole seeds	Several grams daily, or ½ tsp. of the oil, twice daily	A few studies	Improves the nutrition of the prostate gland, reduces inflammation
Willow herb	Teas, tincture	7-12 grams dried herb daily as a light decoction (simmer for 10 minutes); 1 tsp of the tincture twice daily	No studies; empirical and historical results reported.	Reduces inflammation
Goldenrod	Tea, tincture	5-9 grams of the dried flowering tops as an infusion; drink 2 cups daily; to 1 tsp. of the tincture in a little water 2-3 times daily	No studies; empirical and historical results reported	Increases blood circulation to prostate; reduces inflammation

*See Werbach and Murray 1994 for a summary of studies performed on flower pollen for BPH.

Table 2-4. Nettle Root and BPH: Summary of Clinical Trials

Author date	Study type	Preparation & Dose	Number of subjects	Reported Outcome
Belaiche & Lievoux 1991	Open trial	Ethanolic extract	67	Nocturia and other urinary symptoms relieved
Romics 1987	Open trial	Powdered extract	30	Reduced volume of residual urine, increased urinary flow in 50% of cases
Vontobel et al 1985,	Double-blind study	Powdered extract or placebo	50	Highly significant decrease of sex hormone binding globulin in treatment group; improved urine flow volume and maximum flow
Tosch & Müssigang 1979	Open trial	Powdered extract	4,550	Subjective improvement
Barsom & Bettermann 1979	Open trial	Powdered extract (Prostatin)	30	Decreased residual urine as determined by sonography
Schneider et al 1995	Clinical report	Specialized powdered extracts of nettle root and saw palmetto	2,080 patients from 419 urological practices	Subjective improvement of urinary symptoms; less than 1% showed mild side effects
Krzeski et al 1993	Randomized double-blind study	Powdered extracts of nettle root and Pygeum	134	A half-dose worked as well as full dose in reducing nighttime urination and residual volume; side effects were few
Romics & Bach 1990	Randomized double-blind study	Powdered extract	—	Zinc levels were reduced in prostates of treatment group, but not in control group

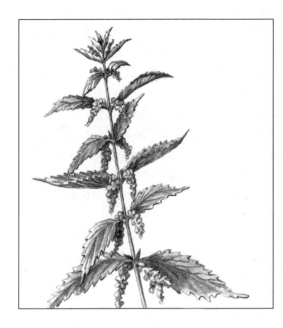

Urtica doica
(stinging nettle)
has shown promise
for the treatment
of BPH in a
number of studies.

that nettle extract alters the binding of male hormones in human blood plasma. The human clinical trials, both controlled and uncontrolled, are summarized in Table 2-4.

The effective daily dose for dried nettle root is about eight to twelve grams, according to the Commission E monograph (Blumenthal 1997). This is equivalent to about four to eight 00-size capsules of the powdered extract daily, two in the morning and two again in the evening, with meals.

Pygeum africanum

Another important botanical extract currently employed in Europe for treatment of prostate disorders, *Pygeum africanum*, shows activity similar to, but stronger than, that of nettle root. In fact, these two herbs are often successfully used together to treat enlarged prostate. In one double-blind study, 134 men, ages 53 to 84, were treated with a combination of the two extracts. Patients receiving either a full dose or a half-dose experienced a significant improvement in urine flow, along with a decrease in urine retention and nocturnal urination (Krzeski et al 1993). See Table 2-3 on page 57 for further details.

In a review of various French clinical studies of *Pygeum* over a twenty-five-year period, a majority of trials shows statistically significant improvement (Andro & Riffaud 1995). Most studies report a complete absence of adverse effects, in contrast with the often debilitating effects of prostate surgery or other Western treatments. An analysis of the pharmacological activity of *Pygeum* shows that it can reduce hyper-reactivity of the bladder and decrease inflammation; some constituents also show anticancer activity [see Mathe et al (1995); see also Werbach and Murray (1994) for a review of European studies that have been performed on this herb].

Unlike nettle root and saw palmetto, there are two drawbacks to *Pygeum* extracts. First, the world's supply of the herb is sold by only one supplier; smaller manufacturers cannot obtain the bulk herb. Secondly, there is some indication that the herb is endangered in its native Africa.

CONCLUSION

Although no final or certain statement can be made about the mechanism of action of saw palmetto extracts at the present time, it is likely that herbalists and physicians alike will keep prescribing the herb, and that patients will continue to benefit from it. By combining this use, human experience, and clinical and laboratory research, we may eventually unlock the secrets of this fascinating plant.

CHAPTER 3

NATURAL CARE OF THE PROSTATE GLAND

Herbs, drugs, and surgery each have a place in treating benign prostatic hyperplasia, but development of healthy habits is probably the best way to create health and relieve symptoms permanently. Paul Bragg, a health crusader from the 1930s to the 1970s, said that a "total program for health" is most effective for eliminating disease.

Developing new, healthy habits to replace old, unhealthy ones takes time and effort, for there is no magic bullet to prevent or cure every ill. Healthy habits, however, are the only true and lasting way to health. Eating sugar daily, for example, without brushing after every meal, will ruin one's teeth in short order; millions of people worldwide have done it. The habits of brushing, flossing, and substituting fresh fruit for refined sugar allow most people to keep their healthy teeth into old age.

Putting forth the effort to establish good health habits is a choice for most people. The easiest way is a childhood that includes these habits, for good health in families is learned as well as inherited. Not everyone, however, is reared with such habits or continues them past the teenage years. Some neglect their health until a crisis occurs, at which point it is sometimes too late to achieve optimum health, although improvements can be made.

NUTRITION AND THE PROSTATE

Good nutrition is as important for prostate health as it is for the rest of the body. No organ or tissue is separate, and none escapes the impact of our daily habits. Everything put into the body and everything that doesn't come out affects health. Generally speaking, a healthy diet is one that has the following elements.

• The diet is enjoyable.

• Taking meals is a relaxed occasion uncluttered by other activities. Food and drink are taken with appreciation of the benefits received. Food is chewed thoroughly.

• About 80 percent of the diet is eaten as whole, natural, unprocessed foods.

• The diet includes a good variety of foods without fixing on any particular food(s).

• The diet includes lots of organically cultivated vegetables, fruits, seeds, nuts, grains, legumes, and a small amount of organic fish and chicken. Red meat can be taken in small amounts once or twice a week for a while in cases of weakness, blood deficiency, and a feeling of being run-down.

• Dairy products are best taken fermented as in yogurt or cultured buttermilk; goat's milk is better than cow's milk; and organic milk is good when available. Whole milk and butter should be kept to a minimum in order to avoid the fats. Dairy should comprise only a small portion of a healthful diet.

- Foods that are low in fat and high in vegetable fiber (both soluble and insoluble) support a healthy prostate.

Zinc and the Prostate

Zinc has long been touted as a mineral that benefits the prostate gland and is essential for its healthy function. While the healthy prostate gland does contain high levels of zinc and may require a good supply to keep healthy, hyperplastic prostate tissue has even higher levels! Consequently, the best mineral support for prostate health may be naturally occurring zinc in adequate quantities rather than purified zinc supplements. The latter should be reserved for use only as part of a complete nutritional supplement that contains copper and other minerals. Fifteen milligrams of zinc is considered a reasonable daily dietary level of the mineral.

Two studies give a little evidence that zinc supplementation may be helpful in reducing symptoms associated with BPH (Fahim et al 1976; Bush et al 1974). In both, the number of patients was small. One group of nineteen patients received 150 milligrams of zinc daily for two months. Fourteen patients experienced a shrinkage of the prostate as demonstrated by rectal, X-ray, and endoscopic examination (Bush et al 1974). The other study showed that zinc supplementation reduced prostate size and helped relieve some symptoms (Fahim et al 1976).

Natural Sources of Zinc

Pumpkin seeds are often recommended as a source of natural zinc. How do they compare with other natural sources? A handful of dried pumpkin seeds (one-third of an ounce or about forty-five seeds) contains about three-fourths of a milligram of zinc. In contrast, one tablespoon of unroasted sesame butter has nearly 1.5 milligrams, a half a cup of wheat bran has a little over two milligrams, and one-quarter cup of wheat germ has 3.5 milligrams. Each of these foods provides more zinc than pumpkin seeds.

Shellfish are the most intensive natural source of zinc. One oyster, for instance, supplies almost the full daily requirement. Oysters are reputed to be aphrodisiacs, and considering that an unhealthy prostate may result in painful ejaculation, perhaps there's something to the old story. Oysters are bottom-feeders, however, and thus may pick up and concentrate heavy metals or other environmental toxins from the ocean floor.

Table 3-1: Dietary Sources of Zinc

Food	Relative Zinc Concentrations	Serving	Approximate percent of daily Zinc
Whole grain products	Whole wheat good, white flour poor; amaranth very good	1/4 cup wheat germ, 1/2 cup wheat bran	15%
Soy products	Tempeh, good; tofu, fair	1/2 cup	10%
Beans	Generally good; aduki best	1/2 cup	13%
Seeds, nuts	Pumpkin highest; others fair-good	1/3 ounce (handful)	5%
Meats	Generally fair; red meat average; fish fair	1 slice	5%
Shellfish	Highest source; oysters excellent	6 medium oysters	500%
Milk products	Fair-good	8 ounces lowfat	5%
Vegetables	Poor-fair	1 cup	2-5%
Fruits	Poor	1 cup	1-2%

Source: Pennington, J. A. T. 1994. Bowes & Church's Food Values of Portions Commonly Used, 16th edition. Philadelphia: J.B. Lippincott Co.

Selenium

Selenium affects proper sperm production and prostate function. Low selenium levels have been linked with depressed immune function and may contribute to prostate problems. Sea vegetables, seaweed, seafood, whole grains, and brewer's yeast are dietary sources of selenium; a reasonable daily intake of the mineral is 50 to 200 milligrams a day. Most whole foods contain a nominal amount of selenium, which helps prevent deficiency (Badmaev et al 1996).

Amino Acids

Amino acid supplements may be helpful in some cases of BPH, but more studies are needed to be sure. There is some indication that a combination of L-glutamic acid, L-alanine, and glycine (two capsules three times daily for two weeks, followed by one capsule, three times daily), might reduce residual urine, nocturia, frequency, urgency, and delayed urination in some BPH patients (Dumrau 1962). However, the number of patients (17-45) was small, the period of the study (several weeks) was short, and upon rectal and X-ray examination, the patients in one group evinced no reduction in prostate size. Urinary symptoms associated with BPH respond well to placebo and psychological factors; perhaps these factors contributed to the positive outcomes of the study.

Fatty Acids

One troublesome aspect of BPH is inflammation; when inflammation is reduced, the prostate improves. Some evidence indicates that maintaining a healthy level of essential fatty acids (linolenic and linoleic acids) and prostaglandin precursors, such as gamma linolenic acid (GLA), helps reduce the chronic inflammation of arthritis (Zurier 1996). This anti-inflammatory action of fatty acids may aid in reducing prostatic inflammation as well.

An excellent source of essential fatty acids is freshly ground flax seed taken daily, perhaps as an additive to cereal or other foods. Sources of GLA include the oils of borage seed and evening primrose seed, widely available in natural products stores. In one clinical trial involving nineteen patients, supplementation with an essential fatty acid complex including linoleic, linolenic, and arachidonic acids seemed to help reduce residual urine in all the patients (Dumrau 1962).

Adding foods that contain fatty acids to the diet aids one's general health and may benefit the prostate gland and possibly reduce symptoms as well. Olive oil, sesame butter, almonds, and sunflower seeds contain fatty acids.

EXERCISE

According to Traditional Chinese Medicine, pain and obstruction develop from a

Table 3-2. Fatty Acid Content of a CO_2 Hypercritical Liposterol Extract of Saw Palmetto		
Fatty Acid	Symbol	Percent of Concentration
Oleic	$C_{18:3}$	31.82
Lauric	$C_{12:0}$	28.64
Myristic	$C_{14:0}$	11.09
Palmitic	$C_{16:0}$	8.89
Linoleic	$C_{18:2}$	5.02
Stearic	$C_{18:0}$	2.70
Capric	$C_{18:0}$	1.76
Caproic	$C_{10:0}$	0.64
Linolenic	$C_{18:3}$	0.59

condition of the body's vital energy known as "stagnation." Stagnation of vital energy, blood, and waste products can occur during times of inactivity, excessive worry, and lack of attention to stretching and maintaining agility. The older one becomes, the easier stagnation can occur. To reduce the effects of aging, exercise and activity is essential because the aging human body has a very low tolerance for sitting around and vegetating.

Both Eastern and Western concepts of natural medicine teach that blood and fluids stagnate in the prostate gland because of too much sitting, causing the gland to become irritated, inflamed, and enlarged. Other contributors to this condition are stress and a high-fat diet.

Exercise plays a crucial role in any program for good health. It tops the list of techniques for coping with physical, emotional,

and mental stress. Gentle stretching before and after more active physical exercising keeps the body flexible and relaxed.

Walking is an excellent form of exercise because it places no great stress on any particular part of the body. Recent research shows that walking can be as effective as more vigorous activities, such as running, in reducing weight, releasing stress, and protecting the heart and blood vessels against disease. Running is also beneficial; it improves circulation and consequently the exchange of nutrients and wastes in all the tissues and organs of the body. To avoid damage to the joints, however, do not run on pavement but on a softer surface such as grass, dirt, or a running track.

SELF-MASSAGE

Massage is one of the oldest and most respected forms of healing. Skilled manipulation of muscles, sinews, and even internal organs, whether by Swedish massage, shiatsu, or another of the many massage forms, creates a wonderfully refreshing and restorative effect. The proper flow of blood and vital energy to the prostate area can be supported by weekly massage. Receiving bodywork is an excellent health investment, but if you just can't afford it, take a class or buy a book, learn massage, and trade sessions with someone with whom you feel comfortable.

Another option is self-massage, which helps maintain relaxation and good energy flow. While there is nothing like a massage from a skilled practitioner, daily practice is often necessary to change old habits of deep tension. By spending fifteen minutes in a quiet and comfortable place, you can use your hands to find out what's going on with your body. Many people are completely unconscious of

where they hold tension and where it hurts, because they never bother to focus on it. As you use massage techniques on your own body, you may discover and remedy areas of tightness, soreness, or swelling that you could otherwise overlook.

Abdominal massage assists the circulation of blood and other bodily fluids in that area, thus indirectly supporting the health of the prostate. Lie on your back and place a pillow or bolster under your knees. Take your shirt off, find a comfortable position, and use a light massage oil if you choose. Place the two hands together, one on top of the other. Begin massaging your lower abdomen with the joined fingertips, using clockwise, circular motions. Then work in a larger clockwise circle, around the navel. Find the sore spots and spend some time "working them out."

You will be surprised that the pain, even if it is strong,

will begin to ease, often after the first session. As your practice progresses, after a week or two, you can really go in deep and work out any tension and pain that you find. Keeping the abdominal area open and relaxed will help improve digestion and can increase energy.

During massage, be aware of breathing. Breathe deeply into the lower abdominal area, then fill the upper chest with air. Hold for a few seconds and release fully. The breath of life is vital to the good health of every cell in the body, including the prostate gland.

Spend three to five minutes massaging the area below the navel and just above the pubic bone. Find any obstructions and tender spots and work them out. Then massage the floor of the pelvis (perineum), which is below the scrotum and above the anus. This is an important area for pro-moting prostate circulation. Try using a good herbal oil with rosemary, lavender, or other herbs to enhance the massage. St. John's wort oil morning and evening as a massage of the pelvic floor may help reduce inflammation; arnica oil can help counteract blood stagnation and relieve pain.

One of the most important steps to healing is knowing oneself. Self-knowledge is advocated by all the great spiritual teachers and healers throughout history. By using our hands to feel what is going on with our bodies, we take a big step towards prostate and total body health.

KEGEL EXERCISES

The average American spends four and a half hours each day watching television. We also sit in the car, sometimes for an hour or two a day, and often spend hours sitting at work. Sitting compresses and restricts blood and energy flow, so it is no wonder that many problems develop in the lower pelvis. That area can become literally starved for oxygen and nutrients.

Regular contraction and relaxation of the lower pelvic region can strongly encourage healing of the prostate gland and bladder. In 1948, Arnold Kegel developed a set of exercises to aid women with urinary incontinence. Today, these "Kegel exercises" are used by both women and men to help relieve symptoms originating in the lower pelvis. Kegel wrote that most people are unaware of the muscles of the lower abdomen; these muscles can be strengthened by regular exercise that also benefits the associated organs (Sandvik 1996). Some studies have confirmed the effectiveness of these exercises in treating stress incontinence, or the involuntary passing of urine during coughing or straining (Burgio 1986;

Hagen et al 1990; Hahn et al 1993).

To do Kegel exercises, begin by sitting comfortably on a straight-backed chair. Put your hand on the perineum, just below the scrotum and just above the anus. Contract the muscles and hold for six to eight seconds. Relax the muscles for the same amount of time. Achieving full contraction of the muscles may take some practice, but eventually you will be able to contract them strongly.

Studies show that one period of maximum contraction and relaxation followed by three or four rapid contractions and relaxations is more effective than a regimen of regular contractions and relaxations. Other studies show that maximum benefit may be achieved with between 40 and 160 contraction cycles per day (Lagro-Hannsen 1989; Jolleys 1989).

Among women who use intensive Kegel exercises,

41 to 85 percent experienced fewer urinary problems than did those in the control group (Sandvik 1996). As with all exercise, start slowly, using up to ten or twenty repetitions for a few days, then slowly increasing the number.

STRESS, SYMPATHETIC TONE, AND BLOOD CIRCULATION

Stress comes in many forms—noise, relationship problems like separation or divorce, exposure to danger, death of a loved one, losing "face," changing jobs, or moving. One's internal thought stream also generates stress when it's focused on something unpleasant, or potentially unpleasant, or the loss of something of value.

Upbringing, genetic makeup, nutrition, and environmental factors influence one's ability to deal with stress, whether it originates externally or internally. Ac-cumulated life experience leads to an ability to cope with stresses that might have been overwhelming at an earlier time; one also learns that uncontrolled and unreleased stress can result in physical illness.

The effects of stress on the inner workings of the body are very complex. Hormone levels, nervous system function, immune system performance, and the actions of internal organs are all influenced by stress. One of the most noticeable effects involves the sympathetic branch of the autonomic (involuntary) nervous system, or the "fight or flight" mechanism.

This ancient system certainly played a role in the survival of the human species; quickly responding to danger by fighting or running for safety determined whether early individuals would live another day. Today, many stimuli or internal feelings can activate the sympathetic system, even when there is little real danger present. Driving a car on the freeway is not without hazards, but the chances of arriving safely are high, despite a few aches and pains from sitting tensely for too long. Yet during this drive the adrenal glands produce more adrenalin than the body and its internal organs need to function well.

Such arousal of the sympathetic system is called "increased sympathetic tone," and it can cause undesired changes in internal functions. The excess adrenalin produced by freeway driving can make a person feel anxious and sweaty. Another function of the fight or flight syndrome prevents blood loss from a fight by restricting blood flow to the vessels on the body's surface and sending more blood to the muscles for action. This is all very well during a fight, but chronic sympathetic arousal, as in sustained stress at work, can result in high blood pressure.

What about the effect of high sympathetic tone on the prostate gland and urinary flow? The prostate gland contracts during stress. A man who already has a problem with urinary flow often experiences a worsening of symptoms under stress. In fact, stress may play a significant role in the development of urinary symptoms, because not all men with enlarged prostate glands experience symptoms. Some men with very little enlargement experience significant urinary symptoms. Perhaps stress is a major determinant of whether an individual will be symptom-free or miserable when the prostate enlarges.

Another effect of sympathetic tone heightened by stress is an increase of metabolic rate—the rate at which calories are burned to produce energy and heat. When under stress, the body produces excess internal heat that can become concentrated in specific internal organs, depending on our individual weaknesses. This is called "pathogenic (disease-causing) heat" in Traditional Chinese Medicine. Some research suggests that BPH may be related to a chronically inflamed prostate gland, just as subtle chronic inflammation in blood vessels can contribute to cardiovascular disease.

Stress Reduction: Meditation and Visualization

In order to reduce stress, it is important to seek habits, relationships, and environments that help develop an inner feeling of poise and peacefulness rather than chaos and turmoil. Two time-honored methods for stress reduction include meditation and visualization.

Although there are various forms of meditation, all share similar objectives of quieting the mind, breaking attachment to personal identity, and helping one become receptive to the influence of a higher wisdom. To meditate, sit quietly, try to shift your mind away from your ordinary stream of thoughts by focusing on the breath or on the repetition of a particular word or phrase (mantra). When focusing on the breath, make sure to practice breathing deeply and fully. This in itself can increase energy and well-being by providing oxygen to all the tissues of the body and helping to eliminate waste products. With continued practice, a wonderfully calming state can be achieved, giving the mind a much-needed rest. Those who meditate regularly enjoy improved moods and increasingly positive outlooks.

Visualization involves forming a clear mental image of what is wanted or needed for the higher good of all. It is based on the belief that if something is imagined often enough, it often manifests, perhaps in a better form than was originally visualized.

Visualization is a healing tool for combating stress. When one breathes deeply and takes a step back from a stressful situation while visualizing a peaceful situation, stress is reduced. A steady focus on a peaceful nurturing scene sustained for even a few minutes can relieve stress and replace it with a sense of poise and calm.

Table 3-3. Prevention of Benign Prostatic Hyperplasia: Summary Chart

Food or Nutrient	Notes	References
Phytosterols	Plant sterols are weak estrogens, can alter metabolism and binding of testosterone.	Buck 1996
Vitamin D	Vitamin D inhibited the growth of benign hyperplastic prostate cells in vitro.	Urinatehl et al 1994; Tomlinson 1994
Animal fats	Weak association with intake of animal fats and BPH-associated urinary obstruction.	Chyou et al 1993
Alcoholic beverages	Moderate use of beer, wine, and sake seemed to reduce the risk of urinary obstruction with BPH; distilled liquors had no benefit.	Chyou et al 1993
Estradiol	Increased levels in men with low testosterone was a positive risk factor for advanced BPH, surgery recommended.	Gann et al 1995
Cadmium	Too much cadmium (a heavy metal) in the diet might be a risk factor for BPH. Sources of dietary cadmium include produce grown with synthetic fertilizers.	Habib et al 1976; Lahtonen 1985

CHAPTER 4

WHAT A DOCTOR WILL DO ABOUT BENIGN PROSTATIC HYPERPLASIA

In the United States, typical treatment of benign prostatic hyperplasia can be medical, using pharmaceutical drugs to alleviate symptoms or to suppress growth of prostatic tissue; surgical, using procedures to destroy and remove the prostate tissue; or supervisory, using watchful waiting in place of active treatment. Until recently, surgery has been the treatment of choice in the United States, and nearly 300,000 prostatectomy surgeries are done each year for the symptoms of BPH (Holtgrewe 1989).

Recently, using drugs to treat mild to moderate BPH has increased and the postponement of surgery is more accepted. Anyone with symptoms of prostatism should be evaluated by a medical practitioner to make sure that his symptoms are indeed those of BPH.

SURGICAL TREATMENT OF BPH

Deciding whether to undergo surgery for treatment of BPH requires caution and a well-informed perspective. Although prostate surgeries are decreasing, such procedures remain second only to cataract surgery in men over the age of 65. Some urologists feel that with expansion of life span, as many as one in four American men with prostate symptoms may eventually undergo prostate surgery.

The potential for unnecessary prostate surgery is great, for these procedures generate more than $2 billion per year (Holtgrewe 1989). An analysis by medical anthropologists indicates that urologists depend on the income from prostate surgery to sustain their practices. The climate of fear created by the medical and drug industries may lead men to undergo unnecessary procedures for symptoms that in other parts of the world are considered quite normal (McDade 1996).

Prostate surgery rates vary greatly from place to place within the United States, although prostatism rates are about the same. In areas with high rates of surgery, life expectancy is not improved. In many individual practices, the rates of surgery cannot be justified by the long-term outcome for patients. To put it

bluntly, prostatectomy is an overused procedure.

If one considers symptom improvement alone, surgery is the most effective treatment for benign prostatic hyperplasia. However, undesirable side effects occur at very high rates. These include impotence and inability to control urine release (dribbling).

In cases with mild to moderate symptoms, a trial of watchful waiting or treatment with herbs or drugs should be attempted, and be aware that watchful waiting is not simply waiting. Symptoms and clinical condition should be periodically reassessed.

Prostatectomy should be reserved for cases that fit the restrictive criteria of severe symptoms. Indications for surgery include repeated blockage of urine flow, even after medical treatment; recurrent infections; bladder stones; and kidney problems caused by obstruction of the urethra.

An especially important factor in the decision making process when considering surgery is how troublesome the symptoms are to the patient. Several quality-of-life or bother-index questionnaires have been developed to help physicians assess the degree to which BPH symptoms interfere with the individual patient's lifestyle.

Surgical Procedures

Numerous types of surgery are used to treat benign prostatic hyperplasia. Some are fairly reliable, but others are considered experimental and lack long-term results. Because of the need for improved treatment options for BPH, and because of the high profits involved, many new procedures are being introduced. The following is a brief synopsis of some of the current ones.

Transurethral resection of the prostate (TURP) is considered "the gold standard"

by a majority of urologists. It is popular partly because most urologists are trained in and experienced with this technique. A wire loop and endoscope (small camera) are inserted through the patient's urethra. The loop is used to scrape away at the prostate tissue with electrocautery, an electric current conducted through a needle or snare to destroy unwanted tissue. This tissue is washed into the bladder and then washed out once the instruments are removed.

The rate of improvement in symptoms is 85 to 95 percent (Carlin 1996). As with all treatments, the rate of adverse effects varies with the skill of the practitioner. A BPH guideline panel puts TURP's postsurgical occurrence of retrograde ejaculation, the ejaculation of semen into the bladder not the urethra, at 73 percent and the rate of impotence at 14 percent. The need for transfusion because of bleeding can vary from 35 percent down to 1 percent (McConnel 1994). There is a 1.5 percent mortality within three months of surgery.

Other side effects of surgery include narrowing of the bladder neck or urethra. One-half to two percent of patients experience TUR-syndrome, neurological and blood-pressure problems caused by absorption of the fluid used to irrigate the bladder.

Transurethral incision of the prostate (TUIP) may be used for patients with a small, fibrous prostate. Instruments are placed in much the same way as with TURP. One or several incisions are made in the gland from the urethra.

The surgery has the effect of relieving pressure on the urethra without cutting out pieces of the prostate. Retrograde ejaculation can be a side effect of this procedure.

Open prostatectomy is an option when prostate enlargement is so severe that operating through the urethra is not practical. An incision is made either above or more often behind the pubic bone to enter the abdominal cavity, and the prostate is removed. This approach is usually successful in relieving symptoms but carries the usual infection and blood-loss risks of any open surgery. Transfusions may be required in up to one-third of operations. Rates of retrograde ejaculation and impotence are slightly higher than with TURP.

Laser prostatectomy, sometimes called VLAP (visual laser ablation of the prostate) or ELAP (endoscopic laser ablation of the prostate), is considered a promising new alternative to TURP (Kabalin 1996). A small scope introduces a fiberoptic probe that applies laser energy to heat and destroy a controlled volume of tissue, which is then absorbed by the body over time. The results seem to be as good as with TURP, and fewer complications occur. Bleeding and TUR-syndrome are eliminated, and much lower rates of retrograde ejaculation and impotence occur. Other complications occasionally do arise. *Transurethral ultrasound-guided laser incision of the prostate*, or TULIP, also employs a surgical laser.

Surgical lasers vary significantly. Currently the most widely available laser is the Neodymium:yttrium-aluminum-garnet (Nd:YAG) which produces tissue coagulation. Holmium (Ho:YAG) lasers, which vaporize tissues, are considered an improved and safer method. Several other procedures use alternative devices to destroy prostate tissue with heat.

Transurethral microwave thermotherapy (TUMT) uses microwave energy to destroy prostate tissue. During this surgery, the urethra is cooled to protect it from damage. Although the procedure is promoted as an effective, safe alternative to TURP (de Wildt 1996), some maintain that its results may be due to denervation (deadening of the nerves) and not relief of obstruction (Ahmed 1996; Nordenstam 1996). A recent review of numerous studies asserts that microwave therapy produces significant subjective and objective improvement and is minimally invasive (de la Rosette 1997).

Transurethral needle ablation (TUNA) of the prostate applies radio-frequency energy through a needle device to produce heat. Though there is little in the literature about the procedure's usefulness, preliminary studies indicate that it may be safe and effective (Millard 1996). Results may not be as dramatic as those resulting from TURP or laser, but complications may be lower.

TUEVP and TVP stand for *transurethral electrova-*

porization of the prostate. These procedures use equipment similar to TURP's, but at power levels sufficient to vaporize the tissue rather than cut it. Results compare favorably with TURP, but with minimal bleeding and no TUR-syndrome (Ekengren 1996). Rates of retrograde ejaculation remain high (Kaplan 1996). This method requires further evaluation; studies are underway.

Balloon dilatation of the prostate is done by inserting a balloon into the prostatic urethra and inflating it to increase the size of the urethra by stretching it. This does produce some improvement in urine flow, but seems to be most effective when the prostate is not very enlarged. Results are mixed, and urine flow shows a tendency to decrease over time. This method is not frequently used.

A *stent* is a metal mesh or wire tube that is inserted into the urethra to keep it open. This technique is used mainly in elderly patients who are considered poor subjects for surgery. Complications are not uncommon; the stent can move out of place, and over time it may become blocked by encrustation.

PHARMACEUTICAL DRUG TREATMENT

Alpha Adrenergic Blockers

The autonomic nervous system controls the activity of involuntary functions of the body, including glandular secretions and the contraction of involuntary (smooth) muscles. There are two parts of the autonomic nervous system, the sympathetic nerves and the parasympathetic nerves.

The sympathetic nerves release the neurotransmitters norepinephrine or epinephrine at their endings. These neurotransmitters then bind to andrenergic receptors on the glands or muscles, stimulating their cells. The prostate gland contains both glandular cells and muscle cells. When the smooth-muscle cells of the prostatic urethra are stimulated, they contract, becoming less relaxed, obstructing the flow of urine, and leading to symptoms associated with benign prostatic hyperplasia.

Pharmacological research has produced drugs to block adrenergic receptors, thereby decreasing the stimulation of the glands and smooth muscles. Adrenergic blocking drugs (Tamulosin, Doxazosin, and Terazosin) decrease the tone of the urethral sphincter and possibly other muscle tissue in the hyperplastic prostate, allowing easier flow of urine. Numerous placebo-controlled studies have demonstrated the effectiveness of adrenergic blockers (Lepor 1992; Brawer 1993; Gillenwater 1995; Lepor 1995). A 1996 study showed typical results: a decrease in symptom scores of 6.1 using Terazosin compared to a decrease of only 2.6 points in placebo (Lepor 1996).

Adrenergic blockers do not decrease the volume of the prostate. Possible side effects include reduced blood pressure, which can cause lightheadedness or dizziness upon standing, tiredness, and a stuffy nose. Use of adrenergic blockers is becoming the first choice of many physicians for treating benign prostatic hyperplasia. The drugs seem to be effective—at lower dose—in relieving what are called the irritative symptoms of BPH: frequency, urgency, and nocturia. Higher doses may be needed to relieve the obstructive symptoms of weak stream and difficulty starting urination (Lepor 1992). Adrenergic drugs are also used to treat hypertension. In some men with impotence due to hypertension, the adrenergic blocker Doxazosin has been shown to alleviate both conditions.

Alpha-Reductase Inhibitors

Prostatic tissue requires the hormone dihydrotestosterone (DHT) for growth. Without the stimulatory effect of this hormone, normal prostate growth cannot take place. DHT is produced in the body by an enzyme called 5α-reductase. Men who are born with a genetic defect that prevents normal formation of 5α-reductase never develop benign prostatic hyperplasia.

This knowledge has led to the development of finasteride (Proscar), a potent inhibitor of 5α-reductase (Steiner 1996). As a treatment option for benign prostatic hyperplasia, finasteride has been the focus of several long-term, placebo-controlled, randomized studies that have shown the

drug to be promising in reducing the size of the prostate gland and reducing urinary obstruction.

In long-term studies using finasteride, peak-flow rates increased and gland size decreased significantly (Tammela 1993; Walsh 1996). In a twelve-month study, patients treated with finasteride experienced progressively decreasing prostate size and reduced symptoms (Stoner 1994). Over a year or two, prostate size may be decreased about 20 percent using the drug, while in placebo groups prostate size increases 8 to 12 percent (Andersen 1996).

However, other studies have shown that changes in obstructive symptoms were not dramatically different than placebo (Gormley 1992; Grino 1994; Nickel 1996). Decreased libido, the most common side effect of finasteride, is usually reported at less than 4 percent, though some studies report impotence rates of 14 percent (Nickel 1996).

WATCHFUL WAITING

A third, nonsurgical option in the treatment of benign prostatic hyperplasia that is growing in popularity with conventional medical practitioners is watchful waiting. Much remains unknown about the natural history of BPH, so predicting the progression and outcome in any individual patient is impossible.

In patients with mild or moderate symptoms of benign prostatic hyperplasia, giving no treatment at all is a viable option. The median probability that an individual's symptoms will improve without treatment is 42 percent. Twenty-six percent will stay the same, and 32 percent will worsen (McConnell 1994). These statistics point out the potential value of natural healing methods such as diet, exercise, and herbal supplements, which are unlikely to stress the body or worsen symptoms, while they can very well improve overall health and reduce symptoms.

REFERENCES

Ahmed, M. et al. 1997. Transurethral microwave thermotherapy (Prostatron version 2.5) compared with transurethral resection of the prostate for the treatment of benign prostatic hyperplasia: A randomized, controlled, parallel study. *British Journal of Urology.* 79(2):181–85.

Aito, K. and E. Iwatsubo. 1972. The conservative treatment of prostatic hypertrophy with Paraprost. *Hinyokika Kiyo.* 18:41–44.

American Health Foundation. 1996. AHF (American Health Foundation) launches nutritional intervention study to combat prostate cancer. *Primary Care and Cancer.* October. 33–34.

Anon. 1993. Hearing explores threats of estrogenic pesticides. *The Nutrition Week.* November 12. 2–3.

Bach, D. and L. Ebeling. 1996. Long-term drug treatment of benign prostatic hyperplasia: Results of a prospective 3-year multicenter study using *Sabal* extract IDS 89. *Phytomedicine.* 3(2):105–11.

Bach, D. and H. Walker. 1982. How important are prostaglandins in the urology of men? *Urology International.* 37:160–71.

Barry, M. J. et al. 1997. The natural history of patients with benign prostatic hyperplasia as diagnosed by North American urologists. *Journal of Urology.* 157(1): 10–15.

Bedalov, G. et al. 1994. Prostatitis in benign prostatic hyperplasia: A histological, bacteriological, and clinical study. *Acta Medica Croatica.* 48(3):105–09.

Berges, R. R. et al. 1995. Randomized, placebo-controlled, double-blind clinical trial of β-sitosterol in patients with benign prostatic hyperplasia. *The Lancet.* 345:1529–32.

Berghuis, J. P. et al. 1996. Psychological and physical factors involved in chronic idiopathic prostatitis. *Psychosomatic Research.* 41(4):313–25.

Berry, S. J. et al. 1984. The development of human benign prostatic hyperplasia with age. *Journal of Urology.* 132(3):474–79.

Blumenthal, M. 1997. *The Commission E Monographs.* Austin, TX: American Botanical Council.

Boccafoschi, C. and S. Annoscia. 1983. Confronto Fra Estratto Di *Serenoa repens* Placebo Mediante Prova Clinica Controlatta In Pazienti Con Adenomatosi Prostatica [*Serenoa repens* extract and placebo in prostatic benign hyperplasia. Clinical results]. *Urologia.* (Italy). 50:6, 257–68.

Braeckman, J. 1994. The extract of *Serenoa repens* in the treatment of benign prostatic hyperplasia: A multicenter open study. *Curr. Ther. Res. Clin. Exp.* 55:7, 776–85.

Brawer, M.K. 1993. Terazosin in the treatment of benign prostatic hyperplasia. *Archives of Family Medicine.* 2:929–35.

Buck, A. C. 1996. Phytotherapy for the prostate. *British Journal of Urology.* 78:325–36.

Burgio, K. L. 1986. The role of biofeedback in Kegel exercise training for stress urinary incontinence. *American Journal of Obstetrics & Gynecology.* 154:58–64.

Bush, I. M. et al. 1974. Zinc and the prostate (presentation). Annual meeting of the American Medical Association, Chicago.

Carlin, B. I. et al. 1996. Transurethral section syndrome. *Contemporary Urology.* 8:13–20.

Carter, H. B. et al. 1992. Longitudinal evaluation of prostate-specific antigen levels in men with and without prostate disease. *Journal of the American Medical Association.* 267:2215–20.

_____. 1997. Percentage of free prostate-specific antigen in sera predicts aggressiveness of prostate cancer a decade before diagnosis. *Urology.* 49(3):379–84.

_____. 1993. Hypothesis: Dietary management may improve survival from nutritionally linked cancers based on analysis of representative cases. *Journal of the American College of Nutrition.* 12(3):209–26.

Catalona, W.J. et al. 1991. Measurement of prostate-specific antigen in serum as a screening test for prostate cancer. *New England Journal of Medicine.* 324:1156–61.

Catalona, W.J. et al. 1995. Evaluation of percentage of free-serum prostate-specific antigen to improve specificity of prostate cancer screening. *Journal of the American Medical Association.* 274:1214–20.

Champault, G. et al. 1984. Medical treatment of prostatic adenoma. Controlled trial: PA 109 vs. placebo in 110 patients. *Annales Urologies.* (Paris) 18(6):407–10.

_____. 1984. A double-blind trial of an extract of the plant *Serenoa repens* in benign prostatic hyperplasia. *British Journal of Clinical Pharmacology.* (England). 18(3), 461–62.

Chyou, P. H. et al. 1993. A prospective study of alcohol, diet, and other lifestyle factors in relation to obstructive uropathy. *Prostate.* 22(3):253–64.

Clarkson, T. B. et al. 1995. Estrogenic soybean, isoflavones, and chronic-disease risk and benefits. *Trends in Endocrinology and Metabolism.* 6:11–16.

Clinton, S. K. et al. 1996. Cis-trans lycopene isomers, carotenoids, and retinol in the human prostate. *Cancer Epidemiology, Biomarkers and Prevention.* 5:823–33.

Coley, C. M. et al. 1997. Early detection of prostate cancer. Part II: Estimating the risks, benefits, and costs. *Annals of Internal Medicine.* 126(6):468–79.

Corradi, G. et al. 1996. Detection of *Chlamydia trachomatis* in the prostate by *in-situ* hybridization and by transmission electron microscopy. *International Journal of Andrology.* 19(2):109–12.

Daviglus, M. L. et al. 1996. Dietary beta-carotene, vitamin C, and risk of prostate cancer: Results from the Western Electric study. *Epidemiology.* 7(5):472–77.

de la Rosette, J. J. 1997. Current status of thermotherapy of the prostate. *Journal of Urology.* 157(2):430–38.

de Wildt, M. J. et al. 1996. High-energy transurethral microwave thermotherapy: A thermoablative treatment for benign prostatic obstruction. *Urology.* 48(3):416–23.

Descotes, J. L. et al. 1995. Placebo controlled evaluation of the efficacy and tolerability of Permixon in benign prostatic hyperplasia after exclusion of placebo responders. *Clinical Drug Invest.* 5:291–97.

DiSilverio, F. et al. 1992. Evidence that *Serenoa repens* extract displays an antiestrogenic activity in prostatic tissue of benign prostatic hypertrophy patients. *European Urology.* (Switzerland) 21 (4):309–14.

Dorgan, J. F. et al. 1996. Effects of dietary fat and fiber on plasma and urine androgens and estrogens in men: A controlled feeding study. *American Journal of Clinical Nutrition.* 64:850–55.

Dumrau, F. 1962. Benign prostatic hyperplasia: Amino acid therapy for symptomatic relief. *American Journal of Geriatrics.* 10:426–30.

Ekengren, J. and R.G. Hahn. 1996. Complications during transurethral vaporization of the prostate. *Urology.* 48(3):424–27.

Emili, E. et al. 1983. Clinical trial of a new drug for treating hypertrophy of the prostate (Permixon). *Urologia.* 50:1042–48.

Fahim, M. et al. 1976. Zinc supplementation reduces the size of the prostate and BPH symptomatology in the majority of patients. *Federal Prococeedings.* 35:361. In Werbach, M. R. 1988. *Nutritional Influences on Illness.* Tarzana, CA: Third Line Press, Inc.

Felter, H. W. and J. U. Lloyd. 1898. *King's American Dispensatory.* Cincinnati: The Ohio Valley Co.

Gann, P. H. et al. 1994. Prospective study of plasma fatty acids and the risk of prostate cancer. *The Journal of the National Cancer Institute.* 86(4):281–86.

_____. 1995. A prospective evaluation of plasma prostate-specific antigen for detection of prostatic cancer. *Journal of the American Medical Association.* 273(4):289–94.

_____. 1995. A prospective study of plasma hormone levels, nonhormonal factors, and development of benign prostatic hyperplasia. *Prostate.* 26(1):40–9.

Garnick, M. B. and W. R. Fair. 1996. Prostate cancer: Emerging concepts. Part II. *Annals of Internal Medicine.* 125(3):205–12.

Garraway, W. M., G. N. Collins, and R. J. Lee. 1991. High prevalence of benign prostatic hypertrophy in the community. *Lancet.* 338:469.

Gillenwater, J. Y. et al. 1995. Doxazosin for the treatment of benign prostatic hyperplasia in patients with mild to moderate essential hypertension: A double-blind, placebo-controlled, dose-response multicenter study. *Journal of Urology.* 154(1):110–15.

Giovannucci, E. et al. 1993. A prospective study of dietary fat and risk of prostate cancer. *Journal of the National Cancer Institute.* 85(19):1571–79.

Gormley, G. J. et al. 1992. The effect of finasteride in men with benign prostatic hyperplasia. *New England Journal of Medicine.* 327(17):1185–91.

Grino, P. and E. Stoner. 1994. Finasteride for the treatment and control of benign prostatic hyperplasia: Summary of Phase III controlled studies. *European Urology.* 25 Suppl. 1:24–8.

Habib, F. K. et al. 1976. Metal-androgen interrelationships in carcinoma and hyperplasia of the human prostate. *Journal of Endocrinology.* 71(1):133–41.

Hagen, R. H., B. Kvarstein, J. Jorgensen, and S. Larsen. 1990. Pelvic floor muscle exercise for the treatment of female stress urinary incontinence. III. Effect of two different degrees of pelvic floor muscle exercises. *Neurorul. Urodyn.* 9:489–502.

Hahn, I. et al. 1993. Long-term results of pelvic floor training in female stress urinary incontence. *British Journal of Urology.* 72:421–27.

Hiermann, A. et al. 1989. The contents of *Sabal* fruits and testing of their anti-inflammatory effect. *Archiv der Pharmazie.* 322(2):111–14.

Holtgrewe, H. L. et al. 1989. Transurethral prostatectomy: Practice aspects of the dominant operation in American urology. *Journal of Urology.* 141:248–53.

Holund, B. 1980. Latent prostatic cancer in a consecutive autopsy series. *Scandinavian Journal of Urology and Nephrology.* 14:29–35.

Hubbard, R. W. et al. 1994. The potential of diet to alter disease processes. *Journal of Nutrition Research.* 14(12)1853–95.

Isaacs, J. T. 1994. Etiology of benign prostatic hyperplasia. *European Urology.* 25, Suppl 1:6–9.

Jacobsen, S. J. et al. 1995. New diagnostic and treatment guidelines for benign prostatic hyperplasia. *Archives of Internal Medicine.* 155:477.

Jolleys, J. V. 1989. Diagnosis and management of female urinary incontinence in general practice. *J.R. Col. Gen. Pract.*39:277–79.

Kabalin, J. N. 1996. Holmium:YAG laser prostatectomy: Results of U.S. pilot study. *Journal of Endourology.* 10(5):453–57. Oct.

Kaplan, S. A. et al. 1997. Pseudodyssynergia (contraction of the external sphincter during voiding) misdiagnosed as chronic nonbacterial prostatitis and the role of biofeedback as a therapeutic option. *Journal of Urology.* 157(6):2234–37.

Kaplan, S. A. and R. P. Santarosa. 1996. Transurethral electrovaporization of the prostate: One-year experience. *Urology.* 48(6):876–81.

Kryprianou, N. et al. 1996. Apoptotic versus proliferative activities in human behign prostatic hyperplasia. *Human Pathology.* 27(7):669–75.

Lagro-Jannsen, T. L. M. et al. 1989. Controlled trial of pelvic floor exercises in the treatment of urinary stress incontinence in general practice. *J. R. Coll. Gen. Pract.* 41:445–49.

Lahtonen, R. 1985. Zinc and cadmium concentrations in whole tissue and in separated epithelium and stroma from human benign prostatic hypertrophic glands. *Prostate.* 6(2):177–83.

Lee, C. et al. 1995. Etiology of benign prostatic hyperplasia. *Urologic Clinics of North America* 22(2):237–46.

Lepor, H. et al.. 1992. Randomized double-blind study comparing the effectiveness of balloon dilation of the prostate and cystoscopy for the treatment of symptomatic benign prostatic hyperplasia. *Journal of Urology.* 147(3):639–44.

Lepor, H. et al. 1996. The efficacy of terazosin, finasteride, or both in benign prostatic hyperplasia. *New England Journal of Medicine.* 335:533–39.

Lloyd, J. U. 1921. *Origin and history of all the Pharmacopeial vegetable drugs, chemicals and preparations.* Cincinnati: The Caxton Press.

Malins, D. C. et al. 1997. Models of DNA structure achieve almost perfect discrimination between normal prostate, benign prostatic hyperplasia (BPH), and adenocarcinoma and have a high potential for predicting BPH and prostate cancer. *Proceedings of the National Academy of Sciences of the United States of America.* 94(1):259–64.

Marchand, L. L. et al. 1994. Animal-fat consumption and prostate cancer: A prospective study in Hawaii. *Epidemiology.* 5(3):276–82.

McConnel, J. D. et al. 1994. Benign prostatic hyperplasia: Diagnosis and treatment. *Clinical Practice Guideline, Number 8. AHCPR Publication No. 94–0582.* Rockville, MD: Agency for Health Care Policy and Research, Public Health Service, U.S. Department of Health and Human Services. February.

Mendosa, R. 1997. Saw palmetto for benign prostatic hyperplasia (BPH). Internet: mendosa@mendosa.com.

Millard, R. J. et al. 1996. A study of the efficacy and safety of transurethral needle ablation (TUNA) treatment for benign prostatic hyperplasia. *Neuro-urology and Urodynamics.* 15(6):619–28; discussion 628–29.

Miller, A. B. et al. 1994. Diet in the etiology of cancer: A review. *European Journal of Cancer.* 30A(2):207–28.

Nickel, J. C. 1995. Practical approach to the management of prostatitis. *Tech. Urol. Fall.* 1(3):162–67.

Nickel. J.C. et al. 1996. Efficacy and safety of finasteride therapy for benign prostatic hyperplasia: Results of a 2-year randomized controlled trial. *Canadian Medical Association Journal.* 155(9):1251–59.

Nordenstam, G. 1996. Effect of transurethral microwave thermotherapy: An evaluation with magnetic resonance imaging. *Acta Radiologica.* 37(6):933–36,

Nordenstam, G. et al. 1996. Transurethral microwave thermotherapy: A comparison between clinical outcome and morphologic effects assessed by urethrography. *Acta Radiologica.* 37(4):524–58.

Ohnishi, K., H. Watanabe, and H. Ohe. 1987. Development of benign prostatic hyperplasia estimated from ultrasonic measurment with long-term follow-up. *Tohoku Journal of Experimental Medicine.* 151:51.

Partin, A. W. and H. B. Carter. 1996. The use of prostate-specific antigen and free/total prostate-specific antigen in the diagnosis of localized prostate cancer. *Urologic Clinics of North America.* 23(4):531–40.

Persson, B. E. et al. 1996. Ameliorative effect of allopurinol on nonbacterial prostatitis: A parallel double-blind controlled study. *Journal of Urology.* 155(3):961–64.

Reece-Smith, H. et al. 1986. The value of Permixon in benign prostatic hypertrophy. *British Journal of Urology.* 58(1):36–40.

Romics, I. et al. 1993. Experience in treating benign prostatic hypertrophy with *Sabal serrulata* for one year. *Int Urol Nephrol*, 25:6, 565–59.

Ross, R. K. and B. E. Henderson. 1994. Do diet and androgens alter prostate cancer risk via a common etiology pathway? *Journal of the National Cancer Institute*. 86(4):252–55.

Sandvik, H. 1996. Treatment of female urinary incontinence: An annotated evaluation of non-surgical therapeutic options. Department of Public Health and Primary Health Care, last updated 16.03.96. http://www.Hogne.Sandvik@isf.uib.no.

Schneider, H. et al. 1993 Treatment of benign prostatic hyperplasia. Results of a treatment study with the phytogenic combination of *Sabal* extract WS 1473 and *Urtica* extract WS 1031 in urologic specialty practices. *Fortschritte der Medizin.* 113(3):37–40.

Schulze, H. et al. 1982. Neue konservative Therapieausaetze bei der benignen Prosntahyperplasie. *Urologe.* A 31:8–13.

Shapiro, E. and H. Lepor. 1995. Pathophysiology of clinical benign prostatic hyperplasia. *Urologic Clinics of North America.* 22(2):285–90.

Shimaya, M. and H. Sugiura. 1970. Double-blind test of PPC for prostatic hyperplasia. *Hinyokika Kiyo.* 16:231–36.

Small, J. K. 1933. *Manual of the southeastern flora.* New York: Author.

Smith, B. 1993. Organic foods versus supermarket foods: Element levels. *Journal of Applied Nutrition.* 45(1):35–39.

Stamey, T. A. et al. 1987. Prostate-specific antigen as a serum marker for adenocarcinoma of the prostate. *New England Journal of Medicine.* 317:909.

Steinmetz, K. A. et al. 1996. Vegetables, fruit, and cancer prevention: A review. *Journal of the American Dietetic Association.* 96:1027–39.

Stoner E. 1994. Three-year safety and efficacy data on the use of finasteride in the treatment of benign prostatic hyperplasia. *Urology.* 43(3):284–94.

Talamini, R. 1992. Diet and prostatic cancer: A case-controlled study in northern Italy. *Nutrition and Cancer.* 8:277–86.

Tammela, T. L. and M. J. Kontturi. 1995. Long-term effects of finasteride on invasive urodynamics and symptoms in the treatment of patients with bladder outflow obstruction due to benign prostatic hyperplasia. *Journal of Urology.* 154(4):1466–69.

Tammela, T. L. J. et al. 1994. Urodynanmic effects of finasteride on the treatment of bladder outlet obstruction due to benign prostatic hyperplasia. *Journal of Urology* March. 149(2):342–44.

Tarayre, J. P. et al. 1983. Action Asni-oedemateuse D'un Extrait Hexanique De Drupes De *Serenoa repens* Bartr. [Anti-edematous action of an hexane extract from *Serenoa repens* Bartr. drupes]. *Annales Pharmaceutiques Francaises.* (France) 41:6, 559–70.

Tasca, A. et al. 1985. Trattamenta Della Sintomatologia Ostruttiva Da Adenoma Prastatico Con Estratto Di Sevenoa Repens. Studio Clinico In Doppio Cieco vs. Placebo [Treatment of obstruction in prostatic adenoma using an extract of *Serenoa repens.* Double-blind clinical test v. placebo] *Minerva Urologica.* (Italy) 37:1, 87–91.

Vacher, P. et al. 1995. The lipidosterolic extract from *Serenoa repens* interferes with prolactin receptor signal. *Journal of Biomedical Science.* (Switzerland) 2(4): 357–65.

Vachon, M. 1996. Cash crop? *Naples (Florida) Daily News.* Sunday, August 25.

Vahlensieck, W. et al. 1993. Benigne postatahyperplasie–behandlung mit sabalfruchtstrakt. *Fortschritte der Medizin.* 111:323–26.

Van Cangh, P. J. et al. 1996. Free to total prostate-specific antigen (PSA) ratio improves the discrimination between prostate cancer and benign prostatic hyperplasia (BPH) in the diagnostic gray zone of 1.8 to 10 ng/mL total PSA. *Urology.* 48(6A Suppl):67–70.

Vogel, V. J. 1970. *American Indian Medicine.* Norman: University of Oklahoma Press.

Walsh, P. C. 1996. Treatment of benign prostatic hyperplasia. *New England Journal of Medicine.* 335:586–87

Wells, T. J. et al. Pelvic muscle exercise for stress urinary incontinence in elderly women. *Journal*

of the American Geriatric Society. 39:785–91.Werbach, M. R. 1988. *Nutritional Influences on Illness.* Tarzana, CA: Third Line Press, Inc.

Wingo P. A. et al. 1995. Cancer statistics. *Ca–A Cancer Journal for Clinicians.* 45:8–30.

Wynder, E. L. and W. R. Fair. 1996. Prostate cancer-nutrition adjunct therapy. *The Journal of Urology.* 156:1364–65.

INDEX